Hormone Fix

LOSE WEIGHT NATURALLY, SLEEP BETTER, INCREASE
PHYSICAL ENERGY AND BE HEALTHY WITH THE KETO
GREEN WAY (90 KETO RECIPES,COOKBOOK,EAT WELL)

By
SUSAN JOHNSON

Contents

INTRODUCTION

Have you been worried about how you can possibly keep your motivation to lose weight and just work on the body you have been longing to get? If so, then it is best that you take on the challenge of trying to lose weight in a week and see how you can finally start changing your physique to slowly work on eliminating stubborn fats in different problem areas. It is true that there are people who would doubt the possibility of losing several pounds a week, but with your perseverance and the proper diet plans and workouts, you are sure to shed a few pounds each week.

If you are one of those people who also doubt the capability of your body to lose weight, then you might want to get the assurance that you can really achieve something every week provided that you would focus on doing all the right things to lose weight. You see, losing weight is not something you can do overnight. It takes a lot of efforts, perseverance, and motivation for you to get the results that you want or even lose a pound or two in a week's time.

Whether you just want to make a weekly achievement of shedding some pounds or just trying to lose some weight prior to attending an important occasion, getting to know some of the effective and safe ways on how to lose weight in a week will surely surprise you. Starting the challenge of losing weight in a week will make you more motivated of sticking with the exercises and diet plans that you had for the first week and continue till you get the great change with your body.

It doesn't matter how much you lose in every week. The fact that you lost some pounds or even a pound is a proof that your efforts are paying off and you are finally in the right path to achieving your dream body. All you have to do is to find out the proper ways on how you can focus on your problem areas and finally shed all those excess pounds you've been carrying for a long time now. Just make sure that you are completely motivated in working on the process and stick on what works best for your body while not compromising your health.

The Keto Green Way

A conventional ketogenic diet is one that is low in (unhealthy) carbs and high in healthy fats and healthy protein. While it burns fat efficiently, there are side effects such as "keto flu," which makes you feel strange, like you have the real flu. And if women stay on a ketogenic diet for too long, their bodies become acidic, creating chronic inflammation that forces the body to hold on to its fat stores.

Now for the secret key: You can start adding more alkaline low carb foods, such as vegetables (especially greens – hence the name Keto-Green) into the diet – foods that make your body more alkaline (a healthy internal state of well-being and metabolic efficiency.) And voila – you'll start dropping weight like crazy and feeling on top of your game – simply by going Keto-Green.

Keto-Green eating naturally manages your body's three most important hormones – insulin, cortisol, and oxytocin, keeping your body in a fat-loss environment. This new, innovative eating pattern is honestly good for men and women of all ages but is the answer for women in the tenacious stages of perimenopause, menopause, and post-menopause:

So, not only did I create what I believe to be the easiest, fun, and enjoyable way to quickly lose stubborn fat… it could very well be the best diet for women.

You see …

- It boosts your metabolism and optimizes your hormones, allowing your body to efficiently burn fat for energy. In fact, it trains your body to burn fat!
- It stabilizes blood sugar and makes you insulin sensitive, so you don't have to worry as much about high blood sugar, weight gain, and various menopausal symptoms—especially hot flashes (one cause of which is insulin resistance).
- It tames hunger pains – no more giving in to cravings.
- It naturally detoxifies your body from pollutants, chemicals, and hormone disruptors that keep you from losing weight.
- It supports the health of practically every organ in your body, including your heart, brain, bones, sexual organs, gut, and skin.

How exactly do you get started on that kind of dramatic weight loss? And what should you eat?

Stock up on Keto-Green foods.

These include eggs, poultry, meat, fatty fish (like salmon and mackerel), low-calorie/high fiber/detoxifying veggies (like broccoli, cauliflower, cabbage, peppers, green beans, asparagus, all types of greens, among others), and healthy fats such as coconut oil, MCT oil, olive oil, nuts and seeds, and avocados.

Start your day with my Basic Keto-Green Shake.

Place 1 scoop of Dr. Anna's Keto-Alkaline® Protein* Shake powder, 1 tablespoon MCT or coconut oil, 2 scoops of my green powdered supplement Mighty Maca® Plus (a great alkalinity booster), and 8 ounces of water. Blend well, and you're good to go!

Shed pounds even faster.

Add a fat-burning, health-building technique called Keto-Green Fasting into your daily routine. It is super-easy, because we practice it already and don't even realize it. It's called sleeping! It involves going without food from dinner the previous night to a later breakfast the next day – a period of about 13 to 15 hours.

Go Keto-Green all day.

For lunch, enjoy a meal such as Lettuce Tacos. Saute together ½ pound free-range ground beef (serves 2); 1 small yellow onion, chopped; 1 tablespoon coconut oil; 2 teaspoons chili powder; and 1 teaspoon salt. Place mixture in large lettuce leaves and top with avocado slices, some chopped cilantro, and diced tomato. Roll up like a burrito and enjoy.

Understanding the Basics of How to Lose Weight

We come across some people who don't gain weight even though they eat whatever they feel like. At the other extreme, there are people, who seem to gain weight no matter how little they eat. Consequently, some remain thin without efforts whereas others struggle hard to avoid gaining weight.

Essentially, our weight depends on the number of calories we consume - how many of those calories we store and how many we burn up. But each of these is influenced by a combination of genetic and environmental factors. The interplay between all these factors begins at the moment of our conception and continues throughout our life.

If we consume more energy (calories) than we expend, we will gain weight. Excess calories are stored throughout our body as fat. Our body stores the fat within specialized fat cells (adipose tissue), which are always present in the body, either by enlarging them or by creating more of them.

In order to lose weight, one would have to create a calorie deficit. A good weekly goal is to lose ½ to 2 pounds per week or approximately 1% body fat every two weeks. The number of calories one eats to accomplish this needs to be approximately 250 to 1000 calories less than one's daily calorie burn. We can do it by increasing daily activities with more daily steps or other non-exercise activities. Standing and pacing burns at least 2-3 times more calories than sitting for the same time period. A deficit of 250 to 1000 calories can also be created by increasing workout time or intensity and by decreasing the food intake of approximately 200 to 300 calories per day.

In spite of our sincere efforts at losing weight, we at times don't succeed due to specific reasons that stand in our way without we even realizing them.

Reasons to Lose Weight

Most people want to lose weight because of the obvious reasons; they want to look better, be more attractive and they don't want to be fat because being fat carries a stigma in our society of being lazy and unattractive. Wherever you look skinny people are idolized in magazines, on TV and on the Internet as being popular, attractive and successful. Everyone wants these qualities because it boosts self-esteem, which is something that people who are overweight battle with on a daily basis. From a very young age right up until adulthood, being overweight comes with a self-consciousness. The 21st century has brought about a health craze, now more than ever people are trying to lose weight. With TV shows like the "Biggest Loser" and "Dance You're A** Off" we are promoting not only losing weight but becoming healthier. There are so many reasons to want to lose weight however the healthier reasons should be closer to the top of the list rather than the aesthetic ones. Use these reasons to motivate you to lose excess weight.

Decrease the Risk of Heart Disease

Excess weight around the abdominal section of the body increases the risk for life threatening diseases such as heart disease. To reduce this risk you need to lose weight, especially around the mid section.

Lower Cholesterol

Being overweight increases your risk of having high LDL bad cholesterol, and low HDL good cholesterol. By losing weight you can lower LDL, lower total cholesterol and improve HDL cholesterol. It can also keep you off cholesterol medications that your doctor may recommend.

Relieve Arthritis Pain

Excess weight puts added pressure on the joints such as the knees and ankles. For people who have arthritis, inflammation in these joints already reduces mobility and function. By losing weight you can reduce the pressure on these joints, which can relieve arthritis pain. It will also improve function in these joints making it easier to move.

Reduce Asthma Symptoms

Although asthma is not caused by extra weight on the body, excess weight can worsen and aggravate asthma symptoms. When your overweight, the respiratory system has to work harder. Excess weight puts a strain on the lungs and adrenal glands, which manage asthma symptoms. Losing weight can reduce asthma symptoms as well as minimize the frequency of their appearance.

Better Breathing

Excess weight puts pressure on the internal organs, which include your lungs. More weight puts strain on the lungs making them have to work harder to breath in oxygen and breath out carbon dioxide. By losing weight, there is less pressure on your lungs making it easier for oxygen and nutrients to be spread throughout the body.

Improve Blood Pressure

Overweight people have double the risk for hypertension (high blood pressure). This is caused because the excess weight puts pressure on the veins, making the heart have to pump harder to push the blood throughout the body. When you lose weight its easier for the blood to circulate throughout the body therefore lowering blood pressure.

Relieve Aches and Pains

Our feet bear all the weight of our entire body. The more weight you have the more stress your feet have to bear on a daily basis. When you lose weight there is less pressure on your feet making it easier to move around and be active.

Better Skin

With every pound of extra weight, the more your skin stretches. As we age the elasticity in your skin declines. Therefore having excess weight as you age will decrease the ability of your skins elasticity. Additionally ones diet can cause changes in ones skin color and elasticity. Overweight people consume larger amounts of carbohydrates and sugars, which causes skin to be paler in color and can increase the amount of skin tags, excess growths of skin on the outside of the body. By reducing these types of foods in ones diet, you can lose weight and also revitalize the skin.

Sleep Sound

People who are overweight have a higher risk for sleep disorders. Excess weight can increase the likelihood of diminished sleep due to sleep apnea. Sleep apnea disrupts sound sleep, which reduces the ability to sleep all the way through the night. By losing weight you can decrease sleep apnea symptoms and sleep all the way through the night.

Decrease Medication

Many medications, prescriptions and OTC medications can be traced back to carrying excess weight on the body. Doctors prescribe all types of medications for people who are overweight such as blood pressure (antihypertensive), cholesterol (statin), insulin for diabetes, and drugs to lower blood sugars. However, by losing weight you can reduce the need for these medications. You can even reverse the effects so medication is no longer needed.

Reverse Type 2 Diabetes

Obesity is a major risk factor for Type 2 Diabetes. Diabetes is the most common disease for people who are overweight. However, you can reverse the effects by losing weight. Weight loss is the most recommended treatment for people who are borderline diabetic. By losing weight you can regulate blood sugar levels and normalize insulin secretion in the body.

Reduced Risk of Cancer

Obesity has been linked to some forms of cancer. Women who are overweight are more prone to have breast cancer, cervical cancer, and ovarian cancer. Men who are overweight are more prone to prostate and colon cancer. By losing weight you reduce the risk for any and all of these cancers.

Increased Endurance and Stamina

With every extra pound added to ones weight, you reduce the ability to do every day activities because you become tired or winded. As these activities become difficult you try to avoid them or find ways around them. However if you lose weight it becomes easier to walk, exercise, climb stairs, etc.

Better Mood

When one is overweight the bodies system is out of balance. This includes the amount of hormones that control mood. Overweight people are at risk for severe depression and most suffer from depressive feelings. Additionally depression can cause one to become overweight because depression reduces the desire to help or prevent themselves from becoming overweight. Losing weight can improve ones overall well being, boosting self-image and self-confidence. Exercise increases the release of endorphins, a hormone that enhances mood, which eliminates depressive feelings. To balance the hormones in the body reduce the amount of fat tissue in the body.

Increase Quality of Life

Overweight people typically suffer from low self esteem, have feelings of shame, and are more socially isolated. Additionally, sexual performance can be compromised by excess weight. When you lose weight you become more confident in yourself. You have confidence in your appearance and you feel better about not only the way you look but also yourself in general. This improves your ability to meet people, gain friends, socialize, and have romantic relationships.

Increase Longevity

Added weight on the body not only increases the risk of disease, but it reduces ones life expectancy. Losing weight can drastically increase the length of ones life. Eating healthier and exercising can increase the longevity of ones life. This includes eliminating and avoiding bad habits.

Reasons for not losing weight

Lack of sleep

Lack of sleep can contribute to weight gain. The experts speculate that sleep deprivation may affect the secretion of cortisol, one of the hormones that regulate appetite. When we're tired due to lack of sleep, we may skip exercise or simply move around less, which means burning fewer calories.

Chronic stress

Stress and weight gain go hand in hand though some of us not aware of this fact. Chronic stress increases the production of cortisol, which not only increases appetite but it can also cause extra fat storage around the abdomen. It causes cravings for foods, which are high in sugar and fat. The so-called comfort foods make us feel better. In addition, we skip workouts because we just feel too stressed out to exercise.

Overeating

The researchers have found that most of us underestimate how much we're eating, especially when we eat out. Careful scrutiny of our diet is the only way to know how much we're really eating. We need to space out our meals in such a way that we don't remain hungry for long. Or else we may overeat at our next meal. We should try eating smaller portions and eat more often.

Exercise

Exercise is another crucial element of weight loss, along with our daily activity levels. If we are not losing weight, we either need to increase our workout time and intensity to match our weight loss goals or need to change our weight loss goals to match what we're actually doing. In order to lose weight, we need to build lean muscle by doing some form of strength training in addition to our cardio. The more muscles our body has, the more fat we'll burn.

Sedentary habits

Any extended sitting such as at a desk, behind a wheel or in front of a screen can be harmful. In addition to exercise, we must try to be as active as we can. We must also limit our screen time. Therefore, we must take a break from sitting every 30 minutes. If we spend more than

8 hours sitting, it could be one more reason we're having trouble losing weight.

Weekend indulgences

Having some treats now and then is fine but indulging mindlessly in treats on weekends will hurt our weight loss goals. The trick is to plan our indulgences so that we can have some fun while staying on track with our weight loss goals.

Unrealistic goals

There are many factors that affect weight loss which again can't always be measured or accounted for with the tools we have. Our body may be making changes that can't yet be measured with a scale or a tape measure. The experts agree that a realistic weight loss goal is to focus on losing about 0.5 to 2 pounds a week. For any more than that, we would have to cut our calories so low that it may not be sustainable. Conversely, we may be losing inches even if we are not losing weight. If we're not getting the results we expect, it's crucial to find out if it's because we're expecting something from our body, which it just can't deliver.

Plateaus

Almost everyone reaches a weight loss plateau at some point. As our body adapts to our workouts, it becomes more efficient at it and, therefore, doesn't expend as many calories doing it. Some common reasons for this include doing the same workouts daily, not eating enough calories and overtraining. We can avoid plateaus by trying something completely different at least once a week and by changing our frequency, intensity, duration, and type of workout.

A medical condition

This is especially important if we're doing everything right and haven't seen any changes at all on the scale or our body after several months. There may be a health problem or some common medications thwarting our efforts at weight loss. One must consult one's doctor to rule out such a possibility.

Tips To Losing Weight Safely

It's the dream of any overweight person to lose weight. The unfortunate thing is that very few people know the right things to do to lose weight safely. To help you out, here are 6 tips to losing weight safely:

Seek Motivation

Let nobody lie to you that it's easy to lose weight. Sometimes you will hit a plateau where you don't lose any weight. You will also encounter some phases where you will be gaining more weight than you are losing.

If you are faint hearted, you will most likely give up. To ensure that you keep on pursuing your dream weight, you need to seek motivation. There are many ways in which you can do this. One of the ways is rewarding yourself whenever you make progress. You should also surround yourself with people who are also interested in losing weight.

Don't Skip Meals

While you should cut on the number of calories that you consume, you shouldn't starve your body. Many people make the mistake of skipping meals in order to reduce the calories that they consume. You should note that when you skip meals, you provoke your body to get into starvation mode thus you have the tendency of experiencing weight gain.

Instead of skipping meals, you should divide your meals into small. To avoid starvation you should take 4-6 small meals a day.

Reduce Sodium Consumption

Sodium causes water retention which causes the weight to stay on your body. To lose weight you should stay away from high sodium foods. As rule of thumb you should stay away from convenience foods as they are usually full of sodium.

Eat Right

The food that you eat is of great importance. As rule of thumb you should avoid foods that have a lot of calories. The best way of avoiding unhealthy foods is ensuring that you prepare the food in your home.

You should also be cautious of the food labels. Before you buy any food, ensure that you have thoroughly gone through the labels and ensure that all the ingredients are in their right proportions.

Exercise

Exercises play a major role in weight loss. They not only increase your rate of metabolism, they also aid in burning fat. Experts recommend that you should engage in 30 minutes to 1 hour exercises for three days a week. For ideal results you should engage in both cardio and strength building exercises.

Set Realistic Goals

It's good to be ambitious; however, you shouldn't be too ambitious. Although, you might be interested in losing weight, you shouldn't expect to lose all the weight within a few days-you should allow the process to be gradual. For example, you should aim at losing 1-2 pounds a day. Aiming to lose more weight than this is not only unhealthy, it's also unachievable thus you end up giving up.

Losing Weight - Factors to Consider

There are many reasons why being overweight is bad for your health. It can, for example, cause or aggravate type 2 diabetes. Obesity is also a risk factor for heart disease and other cardiovascular problems.

So what do you have to do to lose weight?

Eat less and move more is the trite answer usually received by someone who is overweight.

Of course you can lose weight by reducing the food you eat (energy intake) or increasing the amount of exercise you get (energy output).

But the problem of effective weight-loss is much more complex than simply changing the balance between the calories you consume and the calories you expend in your daily activities.

The search for an effective weight-loss formula requires answers to these four questions:

- Does genetics play a role in your weight problems and, if so, what can you do about it?
- How many calories do you need to cut from your diet to lose one pound or kilogram?
- What are the best types of foods (carbs, fats or proteins) to cut for losing weight?

- Is exercise much good in helping you lose weight or for keeping weight off?

How genes affect your weight

Many people do their utmost to lose weight without much success. In particular, once they have lost a few kilos, they find it extremely difficult to keep their weight down... it just rises back up again.

This suggests that the problem is genetic.

In fact, more than 30 genes have been linked to obesity. The one with the strongest link is the fat mass and obesity associated gene (FTO).

The obesity-risk variant of the FTO gene affects one in six of the population. Studies suggest that persons who have this gene are 70% more likely to become obese.

According to research published in the UK in 2013 in the Journal of Clinical Investigation, people with this gene have higher levels of the ghrelin, the hunger hormone, in their blood. This means they start to feel hungry again soon after eating a meal.

In addition, real-time brain imaging shows that the FTO gene variation changes the way the brain responds to ghrelin and images of food in the regions of the brain linked to the control of eating and reward.

These findings explain why people with the obesity-risk variant of the FTO gene eat more and prefer higher calorie foods... even before they become overweight... compared with those with the low-risk version of the gene.

The FTO gene is not the only genetic cause of obesity, which is likely to be due to the sum of several genes working together.

If you have these 'bad' genes, however, you are not necessarily destined to become overweight... but you are more likely to end up obese if you over-eat.

Having these genes also means that you will need to exercise greater discipline over your diet throughout out your life, especially when you have managed to shred a few pounds and want to keep them off.

How many calories should you cut to lose weight?

The big question for dieters has always been... how many calories do I need to cut out of my diet in order to reduce my weight by a set amount, eg one pound or kilogram?

Once upon a time there was a clear-cut answer to this question.

In 1958 Max Wishnofsky, a New York doctor, wrote a paper that summed up everything known at that time about how calories are stored in our bodies. He concluded that, if your weight is being held steady, it would take a deficit of 3,500 calories to lose one pound (454 grams) in weight.

You could create the calorie deficit either by eating less or exercising more (to use up more calories).

For example, if your weight is holding steady on a diet of 2,000 calories a day and you reduce your intake to 1,500 calories a day, you will lose one pound (nearly half a kilo) in one week, ie 52 pounds or 24kg a year.

Alternatively you could burn an extra 500 calories a day (through exercise) to lose the same amounts of weight over the same time periods.

For years, the Wishnofsky rule was accepted as a verified fact. It underpinned a wide variety of diets.

The only problem is that the rule is wrong. It fails to take into account the changes in metabolism that take place when you go on a weight-reducing diet.

The Wishnofsky rule actually works initially. But after a week or two your weight reaches its minimal level, much to the frustration of myriads of dieters, as your metabolism adjusts to the decrease in your body mass and your reduced intake of food.

Until recently there was no way to predict how consuming fewer calories affects the rate at which you will lose weight, especially when your goal is to lose more than just a few pounds or kilograms.

There are now, however, new complex weight-loss formulas that factor in the drop in metabolic rate that occurs over time as body mass decreases. One example is the Body Weight Planner from the National Institute of Diabetes and Kidney and Digestive Diseases in the USA.

What types of foods should you cut to lose weight?

Should you reduce your calories from your fat, carbohydrate or protein intakes? Which will help you lose weight faster?

The numbers of calories in one gram of each of the basic food types are as follows:

Fat... 9 calories per gram

Drinking Alcohol... 7 calories per gram

Proteins... 4 calories per gram

Carbohydrates... 4 calories per gram

Dietary Fibre... 2 calories per gram

As fats contain more than twice as many calories as carbs and proteins, reducing the fats you eat will work twice as quickly as a reduction in either of the other two types of foods, gram for gram.

This is why diets that concentrate on reducing the fat you eat, such as the Beating Diabetes Diet and the Mediterranean Diet are effective in reducing weight.

But if you want to cut your calorie intake by a fixed amount a day (say 500 calories) will it make any difference as to which type of food you cut down on?

For example, will it make any difference to the amount of weight you lose if you cut 55.6 grams of fat (500 calories) or 125g of carbs (500 calories) or 125g of protein (500 calories) from your diet?

The answer is that there is little difference in the amount of weight people lose whether they cut their calories from carbs or fat.

But calories from proteins are different... according to researchers, high-protein diets tend to increase the number of calories you burn. Why this is so is not clear.

However, when people lose weight they lose muscle as well as fat. The more muscle you lose the more your metabolism slows down which reduces the rate at which you lose weight.

Because it preserves muscle, a protein based diet may reduce the rate at which your metabolism slows down.

The problem is that, if you eat too much protein, you could end up damaging your kidneys. The generally accepted recommendation is that you limit your protein intake to a maximum of 35% of your total daily intake of calories.

So, provided you don't eat too much protein, it is best to reduce weight by cutting down on fats (for the sake of your heart etc) and refined carbs that spike blood glucose levels (especially if you have diabetes).

Does exercise help you lose weight or keep it off?

Cutting down on the food you eat is the best way to lose weight. Exercise is less important, at least in the initial stages.

Exercising when you are trying to lose weight can be tricky. It burns calories for sure but not nearly as many as not eating those calories in the first place.

And exercise increases your appetite, so it is easy to eat back on all the calories you burn during an intense work out.

The recommendation, when you are cutting your food intake to lose weight, is to focus on moderate physical activities such as gardening or brisk walking, rather than going to the gym.

But once you have shred those extra pounds and are down to your ideal weight, exercise becomes important for maintaining your weight at its new healthier level.

Top Tips To Lose Weight While On A Budget

One of the top tips to lose weight is to focus on your diet and make better food choices which will not only be healthier for you but which can also help you lose weight. Some people think making healthier food choices is going to cost an arm and a leg and while most unhealthy foods are cheaper, there are still ways to cut corners so that you are able to eat healthy and lose weight without spending too much.

Tips to lose weight on a budget

Say bye bye to junk food

Because most junk food is cheap, most people end up spending a portion of their paycheck on daily or weekly runs to fast food restaurants. This is not only unhealthy but is the fastest way to add pounds to your frame so eliminate junk food starting today but you also need to change your thinking about junk food in order to stop craving it.

While it may seem quick and cheap, the health costs that result from becoming unhealthy from your fast food consumption can be huge including diabetes management costs, high cholesterol management, high blood pressure management, etc.

Anything that increases your risk of developing these diseases should be off the menu. With every bite that you take of fast food, imagine that each bite is getting you closer to developing one or more of the above diseases and conditions.

Junk food is not only available at these restaurants but can be found at grocery stores too, so avoid shopping on an empty stomach and shop alone since children and spouses can pressure you into buying junk food for yourself and for them.

While junk food may seem cheap today, it will cost you so much more in the future when your health is affected so in a sense it is much cheaper to buy healthier foods today since they keep you healthy and help prevent you from developing chronic diseases that are expensive to treat.

Water instead of soft drinks

Choose water instead of sodas or coffee. Water is so much healthier for you. You will not only save money that you would otherwise spend on sodas and coffee, but you will also be healthier. Drinking a glass of water before a meal can help to reduce your hunger pangs which can help to reduce the amount of food you end up eating.

Anytime you feel hungry, instead of reaching for a fattening snack, drink a glass of water and it will help fill up your stomach and make you less hungry which is why drinking 8 to 10 or more eight ounce glasses of water is one of the best tips to lose weight.

Water also helps your body get rid of waste and toxins so drink up to keep your body well hydrated.

It is best to avoid drinking tap water and to avoid the expense of bottled water, simply invest in a water filter. This is an investment you will not regret as it will help you avoid the chlorine and other chemicals present in tap water.

Also fill up on high water content fruits and vegetables such as watermelon, salads, etc.

Fruits and vegetables

Eating more fruits and vegetables is another of the best tips to lose weight fast. Fruits and vegetables not only help you get the essential nutrients that your body needs but they also contain fiber which is the best way to lose weight naturally because fiber helps you feel fuller faster which ensures that you will end up eating less food as well as less in-between meal snacks which leads to weight loss.

It is best to buy in season fruits and vegetables. Farmers markets are great places to buy your fruits and vegetables. You can also buy fruits in bulk and freeze them to prevent them from spoiling and being a waste of money. Wash them thoroughly and dry them before freezing them in plastic zipper bags. Some may need to be peeled and cut up so do so before freezing them. All kinds of fruits can be frozen such as bananas, strawberries, mangoes, papaya, pineapples, berries, etc.

There are so many vegetables that do not cost more than a dollar so in addition to helping you eat healthier, they can also help you lose weight because they are very filling because of their fiber content and have very few calories so you can eat as much as you want. Nutrient rich vegetables that don't cost more than $1 include kale, collard greens, butternut squash, rutabaga, etc. In addition, buy loose fruits and vegetables that you can wash yourself and not pre-packaged and washed fruits and veggies which cost more.

Beans

One of the best tips to lose weight is to incorporate beans into your diet. They not only contain vital nutrients but are an extremely rich source of fiber especially soluble fiber which helps to slow digestion which can not only help prevent diseases like diabetes but which can also help with weight loss. This soluble fiber is not only great for slowing down digestion but is also important to eliminate waste from your body in a timely manner.

Beans are also a great source of protein which is necessary for building lean muscle if you also exercise as building lean muscle is the best way to increase your metabolism which helps to burn more calories. Select dry beans and not canned beans in order to avoid the high sodium content found in most canned beans. Beans are extremely cheap so there is not reason why they should not be in your diet.

To avoid the extreme gas from eating beans, soak the beans overnight first. Dump the water in the morning and add to a pot that you fill with water. Cook for 30 minutes and then dump this water out. Add more water and cook for another thirty minutes and dump this water out for the last time. After this, add more water and continue cooking the beans until done.

Meat and poultry

Limit or avoid consumption of red meat as it contains saturated fats which are bad for your health. Choose poultry instead and if you are on a budget, turkey is one of the cheapest and healthiest poultry choices. Turkey will more than adequately take care of your daily protein needs as well as containing other nutrients.

If you are on a budget, frozen ground turkey is the better alternative to fresh while still containing all the nutrients that you need. In addition, buy boneless poultry that still contains the fat and trim this yourself. You will find that this is cheaper.

Lastly, you will find it cost effective if you purchase meat and poultry products that are close to the "sell by" date and simply freeze them.

Salmon

Another of the best tips to lose weight is to eat more salmon which is also a great alternative to meat. Salmon is extremely healthy for you because it contains omega-3 fatty acids which are not only good for your health and well-being but eating more of these healthy fats can help you body release more of its unhealthy fat reserves which helps with weight loss as well as eliminating belly fat.

Salmon can be expensive but thankfully, canned salmon contains these fatty acids including many other nutrients which makes this a great option for those on a budget who want to eat healthy and still lose weight.

Eggs

Eggs are also another cheap and healthier alternative to meat and egg whites make some of the best weight loss foods. Eggs from free range birds are healthier as these birds were not fed various antibiotics, steroids and many other harmful chemicals that will find their way into the eggs and into your body.

Packaged foods

If you love pasta but still want to lose weight, one of the best tips to lose weight while still eating pasta is to look for Jerusalem artichoke pasta which is low in calories but still high in vitamins and minerals.

Healthier bread choices include looking for those made with whole grains. For hamburger buns, if you buy whole grain buns, this will not only help you eat healthier, but will be a great tool for portion control which will help with weight loss.

Peanut butter

This is not only cheap but is a great source of various nutrients including protein and it is important to note that peanuts are the only complete source of the protein that you will find. You can add them to sandwiches, smoothies, etc. This is also a great healthy snack but do not eat too much because although this is a great source of healthy fats, these fats are present in high amounts in peanuts which will defeat your weight loss goals if you eat too much.

Keto Recipes

Here are some of delicious recipes:

1 Ham and Swiss Crustless Quiche

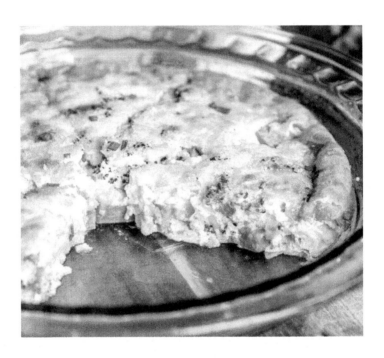

This low-carb Crustless Ham and Cheese Quiche is light and delicious, perfect for breakfast or brunch (or even a light dinner)! Made with a leftover ham or ham steak, broccoli and Swiss Cheese.

Total Time:55 minutes

Prep Time:15 minute

Cook Time:40 minues

6 servings

Ingredients:

- cooking spray
- 1 3/4 cups diced ham steak or leftover ham (9 oz)
- 1 cup chopped steamed broccoli (fresh or frozen)
- 1 cup fresh grated Swiss cheese
- 2/3 cup 2% milk
- 1/4 cup half & half cream
- 5 large eggs
- 1/2 teaspoon kosher salt
- 1/8 teaspoon ground black pepper
- pinch of nutmeg

Instructions

- Preheat the to 350F degrees. Spray a pie dish with oil.
- Evenly spread the broccoli in the dish and top it evenly with the ham.
- Make the custard mixture by whisking together the milk, half and half, eggs, salt, black pepper, and the nutmeg.
- Pour the custard into the dish and top with Swiss Cheese.
- Bake 35 to 40 minutes, until the center is set.
- Cut the quiche into 6 pieces and serve.

Nutrition Info

Calories: 215 calories
Total Fat: 12.5g
Saturated Fat: 6.5g

Cholesterol: 193mg
Sodium: 620mg
Carbohydrates: 5g
Fiber: 1g
Sugar: 2.5g
Protein: 20g

2 Keto Tortillas

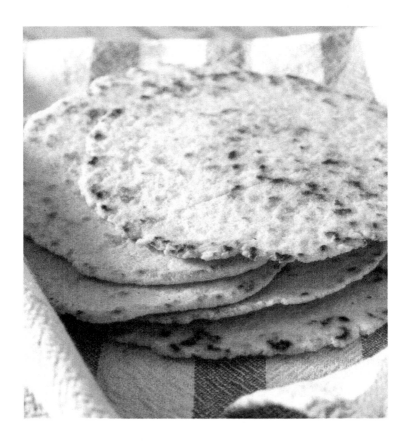

These tasty low-carb and grain-free keto tortillas are perfect for your next taco or fajita night. So easy and quick to make, and they taste like real tortillas!

Prep: 10 m
Cook: 5 m
Total Time: 25 m

Ingredients

- 1 cup blanched almond flour
- 3 tablespoons coconut flour
- 2 teaspoons xanthan gum
- 1 teaspoon baking powder
- 1 pinch salt
- 2 teaspoons apple cider vinegar
- 1 egg
- 3 tablespoons water
- cooking spray

Instructions

- Combine almond flour, coconut flour, xanthan gum, baking powder, and salt in the bowl of a food processor; pulse until well combined. Pour apple cider vinegar into the mixture and blend until smooth. Add egg and water, 1 tablespoon at a time, and blend until a sticky dough ball is formed. Place the dough on a surface sprinkled with almond flour and knead until soft, about 2 minutes. Wrap dough in plastic wrap and let it stand for 10 minutes. Divide dough into 8 equal balls; roll out each ball into a 5-inch disc between two sheets of parchment paper.

- Heat an iron skillet over medium-high heat and grease with cooking spray. Place dough disc in the hot skillet for just 5 seconds; flip it immediately with a spatula, and cook until lightly golden, about 40 seconds. Flip and cook for another 40 seconds.

Nutrition Info

Per Serving: 118 calories; 8.6 g fat; 7.1 g carbohydrates; 4.4 g protein; 20 mg cholesterol; 117 mg sodium.

3 Chicken and Asparagus Lemon Stir Fry

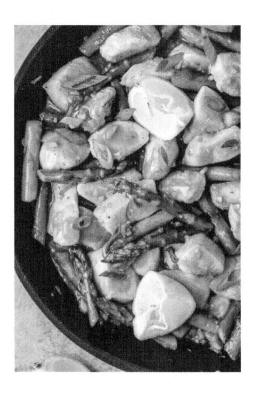

This quick chicken and asparagus stir fry made with chicken breast, fresh lemon, garlic and ginger is the perfect fast weeknight dish.

Total Time:30 minutes
4 servings

Ingredients:

- 1 1/2 pounds skinless chicken breast, cut into 1-inch cubes
- Kosher salt, to taste
- 1/2 cup reduced-sodium chicken broth
- 2 tablespoons reduced-sodium shoyu or soy sauce (Coconut aminos for GF, W30)
- 2 teaspoons cornstarch (arrowroot powder or tapioca starch for whole30)
- 2 tablespoons water
- 1 tbsp canola or grapeseed oil, divided
- 1 bunch asparagus, ends trimmed, cut into 2-inch pieces
- 6 cloves garlic, chopped
- 1 tbsp fresh ginger
- 3 tablespoons fresh lemon juice
- fresh black pepper, to taste

Instructions

- Lightly season the chicken with salt.
- In a small bowl, combine chicken broth and soy sauce.
- In a second small bowl combine the cornstarch and water and mix well to combine.

- Heat a large non-stick wok over medium-high heat, when hot add 1 teaspoon of the oil, then add the asparagus and cook until tender-crisp, about 3 to 4 minutes.
- Add the garlic and ginger and cook until golden, about 1 minute. Set aside.
- Increase the heat to high, then add 1 teaspoon of oil and half of the chicken and cook until browned and cooked through, about 4 minutes on each side.
- Remove and set aside and repeat with the remaining oil and chicken. Set aside.
- Add the soy sauce mixture; bring to a boil and cook about 1-1/2 minutes.
- Add lemon juice and cornstarch mixture and stir well, when it simmers return the chicken and asparagus to the wok and mix well, remove from heat and serve.

Nutrition Info

Calories: 268 calories
Total Fat: 7g
Saturated Fat: g
Cholesterol: 98mg
Sodium: 437mg
Carbohydrates: 10g
Fiber: 3g
Sugar: 0g
Protein: 41g

4 Tomato Salad

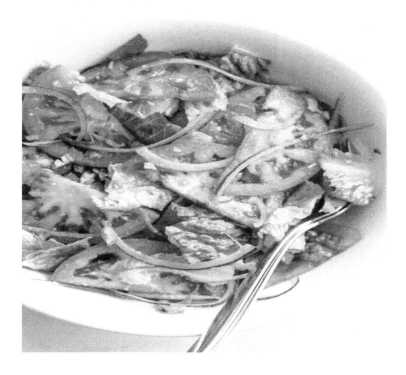

Ripe, end-of-summer garden tomatoes make the best, juiciest tomato salad, perfect served with a rustic loaf of bread!

Total Time:30 minutes
Prep Time:30 minutes
Cook Time:0
4 servings

Ingredients:

- 5 large (8 cups) medium ripe red heirloom or beefsteak tomatoes, cut into 1-inch cubes
- 1/2 cup red onion, chopped
- 8 to 10 fresh basil leaves, chopped
- 1 tablespoon extra virgin olive oil
- 1 clove garlic, minced
- Kosher salt and fresh ground pepper to taste
- good crusty bread, for serving (optional)

Instructions

- In a large bowl combine the tomatoes, red onion, basil, olive oil, garlic and season liberally with salt and pepper.
- Let the tomato mixture sit room temperature for about 20 minutes to let the flavors blend (the juices from the tomatoes will release and create a kind of dressing). Toss well.
- When ready to serve, toss the tomato mixture and divide in 4 bowls. Eat with crusty bread if desired.

Nutrition Info

Calories: 86.5 calories
Total Fat: 4g
Saturated Fat: 0.5g
Cholesterol: 0mg
Sodium: 21.5mg
Carbohydrates: 12.5g

Fiber: 3g
Sugar: 1g
Protein: 2g

5 Basil Chicken and Tomato Salad

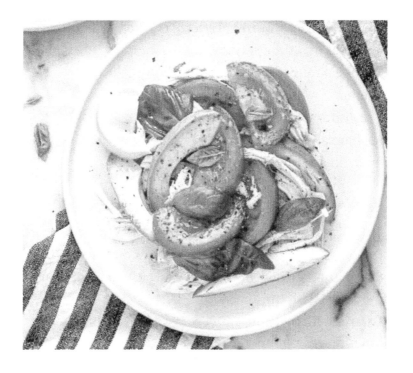

This quick and easy chicken salad is made with the breast meat of a Rotisserie chicken, avocados, fresh tomatoes, basil and lemon juice. Whole30 friendly and a great way to enjoy those end-of-summer garden tomatoes.

Total Time:15 minutes
Prep Time:15 minutes

Cook Time:0

4 servings

Ingredients

- 3 large ripe tomatoes, cut into wedges
- chicken breast from 1 rotisserie chicken (12 ounces)
- 5 ounces avocado, sliced
- 2 tablespoons extra virgin olive oil
- 1 lemon
- 1/2 cup small fresh basil leaves
- kosher salt
- fresh black pepper

Instructions

- Divide the tomatoes between 4 plates or bowls.
- Shred the chicken breast into large pieces and arrange over tomatoes with the avocado.
- Drizzle with olive oil, squeeze with lemon juice and season with salt and fresh pepper, to taste.
- Top with fresh basil.

Nutrition Info

Calories: 255 calories

Total Fat: 15g

Saturated Fat: 2.5g

Cholesterol: 52.5mg

Sodium: 61mg

Carbohydrates: 10.5g

Fiber: 4g

Sugar: 0.5g

Protein: 21.5g

6 Chicken and Avocado Soup

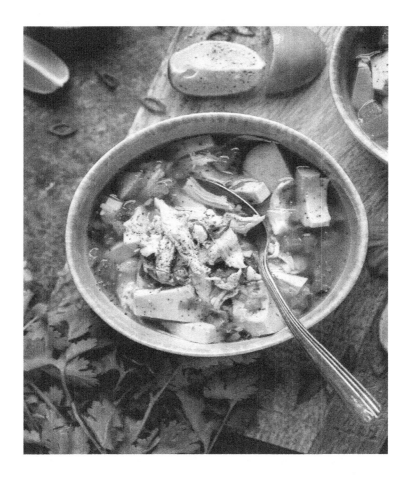

Avocados, chicken, scallions and cilantro in a light broth with a touch of lime. If you are an avocado lover like me, you'll love this soup.

Total Time:25 minutes
Prep Time:5 minutes
Cook Time:20 minutes
4 servings

Ingredients:

- 2 tsp olive oil
- 1-1/2 cups scallions, chopped fine
- 2 cloves garlic, minced
- 1 medium tomato, diced
- 5 cups reduced sodium chicken broth
- 2 cups shredded chicken breast (12 oz)
- 8 ounces (from 2 small) ripe hass avocados, diced
- 1/3 cup chopped cilantro
- 4 lime wedges
- kosher salt and fresh pepper, to taste
- 1/8 teaspoon cumin
- pinch chipotle chile powder (optional)

Instructions

- Heat a large pot over medium heat.
- Add the oil, 1 cup of scallions and garlic. Sauté about 2 to 3 minutes until soft then add the tomatoes and sauté another minute, until soft.

- Add chicken stock, cumin and chile powder and bring to a boil. Simmer, covered on low for about 15 minutes.
- In four bowls, fill each with 1/2 cup chicken, 1/2 avocado, remainder of the scallions, and cilantro. Ladle 1 cup chicken broth over the chicken and serve with a lime wedge.

Nutrition Info

Calories: 297 calories
Total Fat: 14g
Saturated Fat: 2.5g
Cholesterol: 72.5mg
Sodium: 789.5mg
Carbohydrates: 14.5g
Fiber: 7.5g
Sugar: 2.5g
Protein: 31g

7 Cauliflower Rice Chicken Biryani

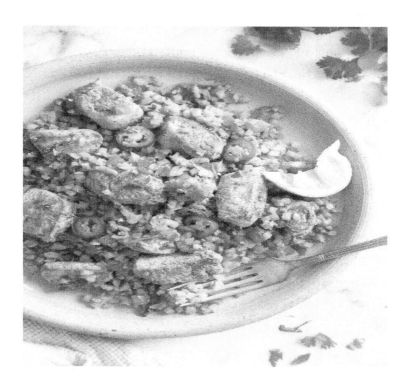

This quick and easy Indian-inspired skillet dish, is a low-carb take on Chicken Biryani, made with riced cauliflower in place of rice.

Total Time:30 minutes
Prep Time:10 minutes
Cook Time:20 minutes
4 servings

Ingredients:

- 1 pound NeverAny! Fresh ABF Chicken Breasts, cut into 1 inch chunks
- 2 teaspoon kosher salt
- 1 teaspoons grated ginger
- 1 teaspoons minced garlic
- 1 teaspoon garam masala
- 3/4 teaspoon ground turmeric
- 1/4 teaspoons chili powder
- 1 tablespoon fresh lemon juice
- 3 teaspoons Carlini Ghee Clarified Butter
- 1 large yellow onion, diced
- 1 to 2 hot green chili pepper, sliced
- 2 packages (6 cups) frozen Season's Choice Plain or Garlic Riced Cauliflower
- 1/4 cup chopped cilantro
- lemon wedges, for serving

Instructions

- Season the chicken with 1 teaspoon salt, ginger, garlic, 1/2 teaspoon garam masala, chili powder, 1/4 teaspoon turmeric and lemon juice.
- In a large skillet over high heat, add 1 teaspoon ghee. Add half of the chicken and cook until browned, and cooked through, about 5 minutes stirring halfway.
- Set aside and repeat with the remaining ghee and chicken. Set aside.

- Add 2 teaspoons ghee to the skillet, reduce heat to medium-high and add the onion, cook until they become golden about 3 to 4 minutes.
- Add the green chili, cauliflower rice, remaining 1 teaspoon of salt, 1/2 teaspoon garam masala and 1/2 teaspoon turmeric.
- Cook, stirring until tender, about 6 minutes.
- Stir in chicken and garnish with cilantro.
- Serve with lemon wedges.

Nutrition Info

Calories: 221 calories

Total Fat: 6.5g

Saturated Fat: 3g

Cholesterol: 92mg

Sodium: 646mg

Carbohydrates: 11.5g

Fiber: 4g

Sugar: 5.5g

Protein: 30g

8 Meal Prep Taco Salad

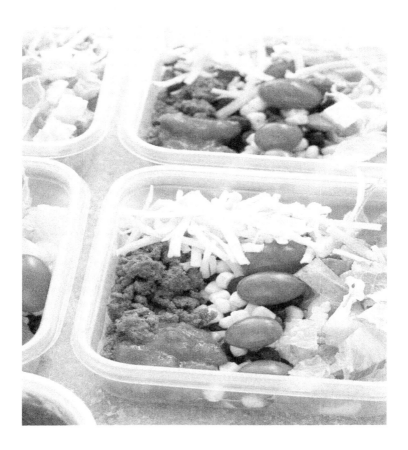

Total Time:30 minutes
Prep Time:10 minutes
Cook Time:20 minutes
4 servings

Ingredients:

Dressing:

- 1/2 cup jarred mild salsa
- 4 teaspoons extra virgin olive oil
- juice of 1/2 lime

Meat:

- 1 lb 93% ground turkey
- 1 teaspoon garlic powder
- 1 teaspoon cumin
- 1 teaspoon kosher salt
- 1/2 teaspoon chili powder
- 1/2 teaspoon paprika
- 1/2 teaspoon oregano
- 1/2 small onion, minced
- 2 tablespoons bell pepper, minced
- 1/2 cup water
- 4 ounces canned tomato sauce (1/2 can)

For the Salad:

- 6 cups chopped romaine lettuce
- 1 cup pico de gallo
- 1/2 cup shredded cheddar
- 4 lime wedges, for serving
- (optional) greek yogurt or sour cream

Instructions

- Brown the turkey in a large skillet breaking it into smaller pieces as it cooks.
- When no longer pink add dry seasoning and mix well.
- Add the onion, pepper, water and tomato sauce and cover.
- Simmer on low for about 20 minutes.
- Divide the meat equally between the 4 meal prep containers.
- Meanwhile, while the meat is cooking, make the dressing: combine the salsa, olive oil and lime juice; transfer to 4 small containers.
- Divide the lettuce in 4 ziplock bags.
- Divide pico de gallo, sour cream or yogurt, if using and cheese in small containers. Cover and refrigerate.
- To serve, remove the lettuce and containers, heat the meat then make a salad by placing the lettuce in a bowl or plate.
- Top with the meat, pico de gallo, cheese and finish with dressing.

Nutrition Info

Calories: 312 calories

Total Fat: 17.5g

Saturated Fat: 5.5g

Cholesterol: 92.5mg

Sodium: 905mg

Carbohydrates: 13g

Fiber: 4g

Sugar: 5.5g

Protein: 28.5g

9 Air Fryer Turkey Breast

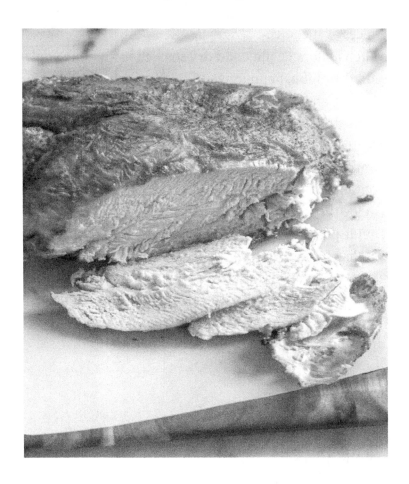

Roasting a turkey breast in the air fryer yields perfectly cooked, moist and juicy meat on the inside with a beautiful deep golden brown skin.

Total Time:1 hour

Prep Time:5 minutes

Cook Time:55 minutes

10 servings

Ingredients:

- 4 pound turkey breast, on the bone with skin (ribs removed)
- 1 tablespoon olive oil
- 2 teaspoons kosher
- 1/2 tablespoon dry turkey or poultry seasoning (I used Bell's which has not salt)

Instructions

- Rub 1/2 tablespoon of oil all over the turkey breast. Season both sides with salt and turkey seasoning then rub in the remaining half tablespoon of oil over the skin side.
- Preheat the air fryer 350F and cook skin side down 20 minutes, turn over and cook until the internal temperature is 160F using an instant-read thermometer about 30 to 40 minutes more depending on the size of your breast. Let is rest 10 minutes before carving.

Nutrition Info

Calories: 226 calories

Total Fat: 10g

Saturated Fat: 2.5g

Cholesterol: 84mg

Sodium: 296mg

Carbohydrates: 0g

Fiber: 0g

Sugar: 0g

Protein: 32.5g

10 Air Fryer Bacon Wrapped Chicken Bites

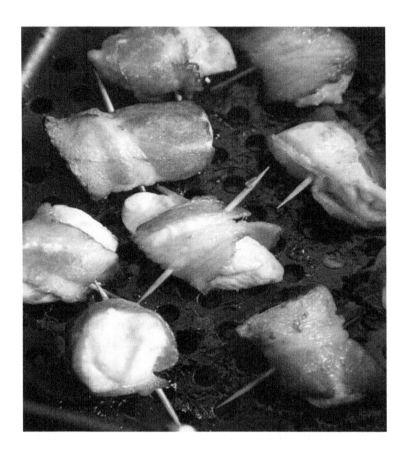

Bacon wrapped chicken bites are the easiest appetizer, made with just TWO ingredients. Using the air fryer, the bacon comes out crisp on the outside, and the chicken juicy and tender inside.

Total Time:18 minutes
Prep Time:10 minutes
Cook Time:8 minutes
10 servings

Ingredients:

- 1.25 lbs (3) boneless skinless chicken breast, cut in 1-inch chunks (about 30 pieces)
- 10 slices center cut bacon, cut into thirds
- optional, duck sauce or Thai sweet chili sauce for dipping

Instructions

- Preheat the air fryer.
- Wrap a piece of bacon around each piece of chicken and secure with a toothpick.
- Air fry, in batches in an even layer 400F for 8 minutes, turning halfway until the chicken is cooked and the bacon is browned.
- Blot on a paper towel and serve right away.

Nutrition Info

Calories: 98 calories

Total Fat: 3.5g

Saturated Fat: 1g

Cholesterol: 44mg

Sodium: 130.5mg

Carbohydrates: 0g

Fiber: 0g

Sugar: 0g

Protein: 16g

11 Roasted Salmon with Fresh Herbs

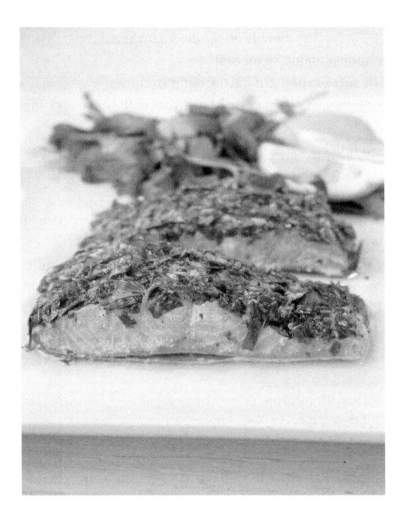

This simple, healthy Baked Salmon dish is made with fresh lemon, and lots of fresh herbs such as dill, parsley, chives.

Total Time:25 minutes

Prep Time:5 minutes

Cook Time:20 minutes

Ingredients:

- 2 lemons
- 8 to 10 parsley sprigs
- extra virgin olive oil
- 1 whole skin-on side of wild salmon, such as sockeye or coho, about 2 pounds
- 1/2 teaspoon kosher salt
- fresh black pepper, to taste
- 2 tablespoons chopped fresh dill
- 1 tablespoons chopped fresh chives
- 1 tablespoons chopped fresh parsley

Instructions

- Slice 1 of the lemons thin, the second into wedges.
- Place the lemon slices on a large sheet pan arranged in the center just under the fish.
- Top with parsley sprigs and drizzle with 1 teaspoon of olive oil.
- Drizzle the remaining 1 teaspoon of olive oil over the flesh side of the fish and rub all over, season with salt and pepper.
- Transfer to the pan over the lemon slices, skin side down.
- Preheat the oven to 450F.
- Roast 15 to 20 minutes, depending on the thickness of the fish, until the thickest part of the fish is cooked though in the center.
- Top with fresh herbs and serve with lemon wedges.

Nutrition Info

Calories: 233 calories

Total Fat: 11g

Saturated Fat: 1.5g

Cholesterol: 83mg

Sodium: 160mg

Carbohydrates: 2g

Fiber: 1g

Sugar: 0g

Protein: 30.5g

12 Huevos Pericos (Colombian Scrambled Eggs)

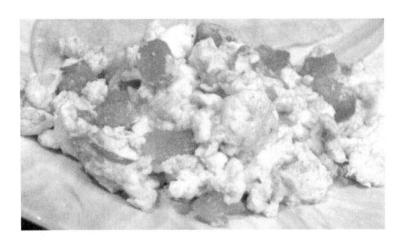

This Colombian classic breakfast dish known as Huevos Pericos made with eggs, scallions and tomatoes is one of my favorite ways to prepare eggs.

Total Time:10 minutes
Prep Time:2 minutes
Cook Time:8 minutes
2 servings

Ingredients:

- 2 teaspoons olive oil
- 3 to 4 medium scallions, white and green parts, sliced thin
- 1 medium roma or vine tomato, seeded and diced
- 6 large eggs, beaten with fork
- kosher salt or adobo seasoning salt

Instructions

- Heat olive oil in a medium nonstick skillet over medium heat.
- Add the scallions and cook until they soften, about 3 to 4 minutes.
- Add the tomato and season with adobo or salt, cook until the liquid from the tomato evaporates, about 3 to 4 minutes.
- Add the beaten eggs to pan with more adobo or salt to taste and cook over medium heat, stirring a few times until just cooked.

Nutrition Info

Calories: 272 calories
Total Fat: 19g
Saturated Fat: 5.5g
Cholesterol: 558mg

Sodium: 220.5mg

Carbohydrates: 5g

Fiber: 1g

Sugar: 1.5g

Protein: 19.5g

13 Instant Pot Deviled Eggs

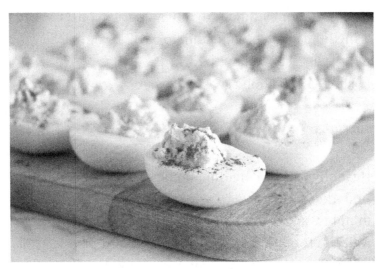

When it comes to making deviled eggs, I keep my ingredients pretty classic, but I love adding little pickle juice to my the yolks for a pop of flavor! Making hard boiled eggs in the Instant Pot will give you perfect, easier to peel eggs every time.

Total Time:30 mminutes

Prep Time:15 minutes

Cook Time:15 minutes

6 servings

Ingredients:

- 6 large eggs
- 1 cup water
- rack that comes with the Instant Pot
- 2 tablespoons mayonaisse
- 1 tablespoon 2% milk
- 1 teaspoon dill pickle juice
- 1/8 teaspoon salt
- fresh black pepper, to taste
- paprika for sprinkling
- fresh dill, for garnish

Instructions

- Place the rack in the bottom of the pot. Pour the water in the pot. Place the eggs on the rack.
- High pressure on manual 5 minutes.
- Natural release 5 minutes then use quick release, then quickly run the eggs under cold running water until cool enough to hold.
- Peel the eggs and slice in half lengthwise. Remove yolks and transfer to a medium-sized bowl.
- Add the mayo, milk, pickle juice, salt, pepper then use a fork to mash well.
- Spoon filling into each egg white. Sprinkle with paprika, dill and serve.

Nutrition Info

Calories: 104 calories

Total Fat: 8g

Saturated Fat: 2g

Cholesterol: 187.5mg

Sodium: 119mg

Carbohydrates: 0.5g

Fiber: 0g

Sugar: 1g

Protein: 6.5g

14 Cream of Asparagus Soup

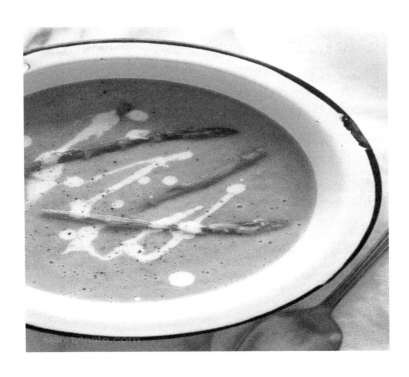

It's pure comfort in a bowl and so simple to make. This recipe is made with just 5 ingredients, not counting salt and pepper and is ready under 25 minutes!

Total Time:25 minutes
6 servings

Ingredients:

- 2 lbs asparagus (2 bunches), tough ends snapped off
- 1 tbsp unsalted butter
- 1 medium onion, chopped
- 6 cups reduced sodium chicken broth
- 2 tbsp low fat sour cream
- kosher salt and fresh pepper, to taste

Instructions

- Melt butter over low heat in a large pot. Add onion and sauté until soft, about 2-minutes.
- Cut the asparagus in half and add to the pot along with chicken broth and black pepper, to taste. Bring to a boil, cover and cook low about 20 minutes or until asparagus is very tender.
- Remove from heat, add sour cream and using your hand held blender, puree until smooth (or in two batches in a large blender).

Nutrition Info

Calories: 81 calories

Total Fat: 3g

Saturated Fat: 2g

Cholesterol: 7mg

Sodium: 576mg

Carbohydrates: 10g

Fiber: 4g

Sugar: 1g

Protein: 6g

15 Instant Pot Corned Beef and Cabbage

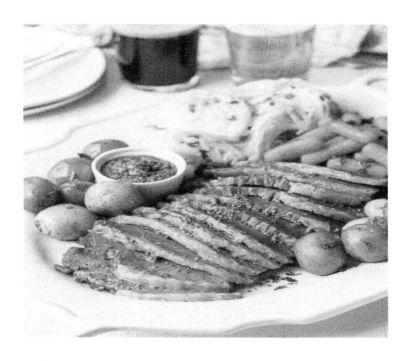

This easy Instant Pot Corned Beef and Cabbage recipe, made with beef brisket, cabbage and carrots comes out so tender and delicious!

Total Time:1 hour 45 minutes
Prep Time:5 minutes
Cook Time:1 hour 35 minutes
6 servings

Ingredients:

- 2 pounds trimmed, lean corned beef brisket
- 3 medium carrots, peeled and cut into 1-inch chunks
- 1 cup frozen pearl onions
- 1/4 cup chopped fresh parsley
- 2 bay leaves
- 1/8 tsp whole peppercorns
- 1 medium head cabbage, cut into 6 wedges

Instructions

- Place the corned beef brisket, carrots, pearl onions, parsley, bay leaves and peppercorns in the Instant pot and add 3 cups of water.
- Cover and cook on high pressure 1 1/2 hours. Natural release then open.
- Add the cabbage to the top, cover and cook on high pressure 3 minutes, quick release.
- Remove meat and slice into 6 pieces.

Nutrition Info

Calories: 359.5 calories

Total Fat: 23g

Saturated Fat: 7g

Cholesterol: 81.5mg

Sodium: 1892mg

Carbohydrates: 13g

Fiber: 5g

Sugar: 7g

Protein: 25g

16 Perfect Hard Boiled Eggs Every Time

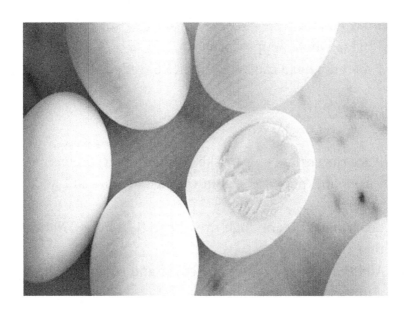

Having hard boiled eggs on hand for quick breakfast on the go or to add to salads and sandwiches makes busy weekdays so much easier. This foolproof stove top method for boiling eggs every time.

Total Time:25 minutes
Prep Time:5 minutes
Cook Time:20 minutes
4 Servings

Ingredients:

- 4 large eggs with no cracks
- enough water to cover eggs

Instructions

- Place the eggs in a medium pan, and cover with about an inch of cold water.
- Turn heat on to medium and bring the water to a boil. When the water boils, shut the flame off and cover for 20 minutes, the steam will cook them. Run under cold water to let the eggs cool, then peel.

Nutrition Info

Calories: 77 calories
Total Fat: 5g
Saturated Fat: 2g
Cholesterol: 212mg

Sodium: 62mg

Carbohydrates: 1g

Fiber: 0g

Sugar: 1g

Protein: 6g

17 Green Bean Salad

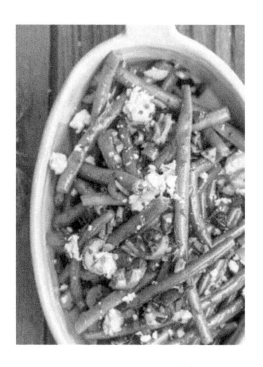

One of my favorite ways to enjoy green beans–in a chilled green bean salad recipe! The delicious flavors of these balsamic green beans made with black olives, scallions and eggs complement any meal or holiday potluck.

Total Time:20 minutes
Prep Time:10 minutes
Cook Time:10 minutes
6 servings

Ingredients:

- 24 oz (6 cups) string beans beans, ends trimmed
- 2.25 ounce can sliced black olives, drained (check labels for Whole30)
- 3 tablespoons balsamic vinegar
- 3 tablespoons extra virgin olive oil
- 3 medium scallions, chopped
- 3/4 teaspoon kosher salt
- fresh black pepper, to taste
- 5 hard boiled eggs, peeled and sliced

Instructions

- Place green beans in a large pot and cover with water, about 6 cups. Bring to a boil, then cover and cook until tender crisp, about 6 minutes (don't overcook or they will get mushy).
- Drain and rinse under cold water when done to prevent them from overcooking, drain.
- In a large bowl, combine balsamic, oil, salt and pepper. Toss in the green beans, scallions and olives.
- Mix well and top with sliced eggs. Refrigerate and serve chilled or room temperature.

Nutrition Info

Calories: 176 calories

Total Fat: 12g

Saturated Fat: 2.5g

Cholesterol: 155mg

Sodium: 308mg

Carbohydrates: 11g

Fiber: 4.5g

Sugar: 4g

Protein: 7.5g

18 Chicken and Asparagus Lemon Stir Fry

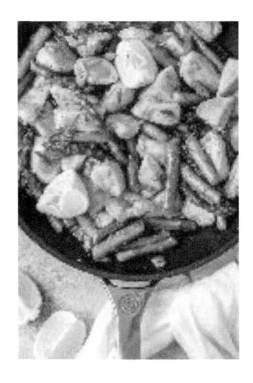

This quick chicken and asparagus stir fry made with chicken breast, fresh lemon, garlic and ginger is the perfect fast weeknight dish.

Total Time:30 minutes
4 servings

Ingredients:

- 1 1/2 pounds skinless chicken breast, cut into 1-inch cubes
- Kosher salt, to taste
- 1/2 cup reduced-sodium chicken broth
- 2 tablespoons reduced-sodium shoyu or soy sauce (Coconut aminos for GF, W30)
- 2 teaspoons cornstarch (arrowroot powder or tapioca starch for whole30)
- 2 tablespoons water
- 1 tbsp canola or grapeseed oil, divided
- 1 bunch asparagus, ends trimmed, cut into 2-inch pieces
- 6 cloves garlic, chopped
- 1 tbsp fresh ginger
- 3 tablespoons fresh lemon juice
- fresh black pepper, to taste

Instructions

- Lightly season the chicken with salt.
- In a small bowl, combine chicken broth and soy sauce.
- In a second small bowl combine the cornstarch and water and mix well to combine.

- Heat a large non-stick wok over medium-high heat, when hot add 1 teaspoon of the oil, then add the asparagus and cook until tender-crisp, about 3 to 4 minutes.
- Add the garlic and ginger and cook until golden, about 1 minute. Set aside.
- Increase the heat to high, then add 1 teaspoon of oil and half of the chicken and cook until browned and cooked through, about 4 minutes on each side.
- Remove and set aside and repeat with the remaining oil and chicken. Set aside.
- Add the soy sauce mixture; bring to a boil and cook about 1-1/2 minutes.
- Add lemon juice and cornstarch mixture and stir well, when it simmers return the chicken and asparagus to the wok and mix well, remove from heat and serve.

Nutrition Info

Calories: 268 calories
Total Fat: 7g
Saturated Fat: g
Cholesterol: 98mg
Sodium: 437mg
Carbohydrates: 10g
Fiber: 3g
Sugar: 0g
Protein: 41g

19 Instant Pot Bolognese

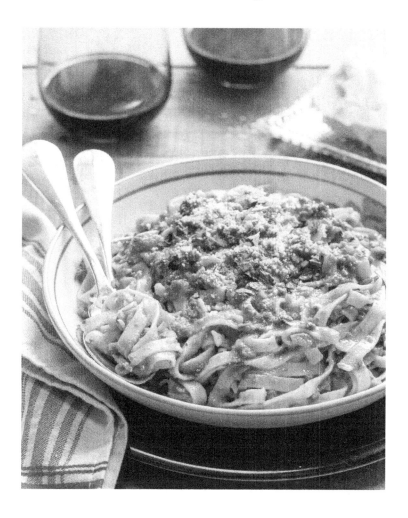

This is the best Bolognese sauce recipe, a staple in my home. It's so easy to make, I always make a big batch for dinner and freeze the rest to use throughout the month – a huge time saver! Making it in the pressure cooker makes this Sunday sauce a dish you can whip up any night of the week!

Total Time:60 minutes

Prep Time:15 minutes

Cook Time:45 minutes

10 servings

Ingredients:

- 4 ounces pancetta (or center cut bacon), chopped
- 1 tablespoon unsalted butter
- 1 large white onion, minced
- 2 celery stalks (about 3/4 cup), minced
- 2 carrots (about 3/4 cup), minced
- 2 lb lean ground beef
- 1/4 cup dry white wine, such as Pinot Grigio
- 2 (28 oz) cans crushed tomatoes (I love Tuttorosso)
- 3 bay leaves
- 1/2 teaspoon kosher salt and fresh black pepper, to taste
- 1/2 cup half & half cream
- 1/4 cup chopped fresh parsley

Instructions

- Press saute on the Instant Pot, sauté the pancetta over low heat until the fat melts, about 4-5 minutes.
- Add the butter, onion, celery and carrots and cook until soft, about 6 to 8 minutes.
- Add the meat and season it with 3/4 teaspoons salt and black pepper to taste and sauté until browned, about 4 to 5 minutes,

breaking the meat up into smaller pieces with a wooden spoon as it cooks.

- Add the wine and cook until it reduces down, about 3-4 minutes.
- Add crushed tomatoes, bay leaves, 3/4 teaspoon salt and fresh cracked black pepper; cover and cook high pressure 15 minutes.
- Natural release, stir in the half & half and garnish with parsley; serve over your favorite pasta, zucchini noodles or spaghetti squash.

Nutrition Info

Calories: 191 calories

Total Fat: 8.5g

Saturated Fat: 4g

Cholesterol: 124mg

Sodium: 568mg

Carbohydrates: 12.5g

Fiber: 0.5g

Sugar: 6.5g

Protein: 12g

20 Sautéed Brussels Sprouts with Pancetta

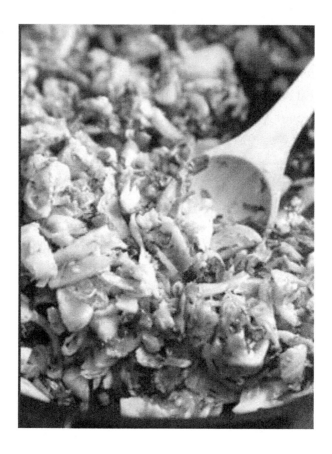

Sautéed Brussels Sprouts with Pancetta is the best Brussel sprout recipe! Lightly pan fried until crisp and slightly browned on the edges, it's my favorite way to cook and eat them!

Total Time:20 minutes
Prep Time:10 minutes
Cook Time:10 minutes
9 servings

Ingredients:

- 2 oz pancetta, minced
- 2 lb brussels sprouts (weight after outer leaves and stems removed)
- 1.5 tbsp extra virgin olive oil
- 4 cloves garlic, minced or sliced thin
- kosher salt and fresh ground pepper

Instructions

- With a large sharp knife, finely shred the brussels sprouts after thoroughly washing.
- In a deep heavy saute pan, sauté pancetta on medium-low heat until fat melts and pancetta becomes golden, about 5 minutes. Add olive oil and garlic and sauté until golden. Add shredded brussels sprouts, salt and pepper to taste and sauté on high heat for about 6 to 10 minutes, until tender crisp.
- Makes about 7 cups.

Nutrition Info

Calories: 87 calories
Total Fat: 4g
Saturated Fat: 1g
Cholesterol: 0mg
Sodium: 148mg
Carbohydrates: 9.5g
Fiber: 4g

Sugar: 3.5g

Protein: 3.5g

21 Tuna Salad Deviled Eggs

These Tuna Stuffed Deviled Eggs are perfect to pack for lunch or serve as an appetizer!

Total Time:20 minutes

Prep Time:20 minutes

Cook Time:0 minutes

4 servings

Ingredients:

- 8 large hard boiled eggs, halved (Instant Pot hard boiled egg recipe here)
- 2 (6 oz) cans albacore tuna, packed in water, drained
- 1 tbsp red onion, minced
- 1/3 cup light mayo (use compliant mayo for whole30)
- 1 teaspoon red wine vinegar
- chopped fresh chives
- salt and pepper, to taste

Instructions

- In a medium bowl combine the egg yolks with mayo and mash.
- Add tuna, red onion and red wine vinegar.

- Scoop heaping spoonfuls of the tuna salad into the 16 halved eggs. Garnish with chives.

Nutrition Info

Calories: 264 calories
Total Fat: 16g
Saturated Fat: 3.5g
Cholesterol: 397mg
Sodium: 472mg
Carbohydrates: 3g
Fiber: 0g
Sugar: 1g
Protein: 26.5g

22 Smoked Salmon Pinwheels

These elegant smoked salmon pinwheels are perfect if you want to enjoy lox without the bagels for a low-carb, keto appetizer.

Total Time:20 minutes
4 servings

Ingredients:

- 8 ounces thinly sliced cold smoked salmon (I like Nova Lox)
- 4 ounces 1/3 less fat cream cheese
- 1/4 medium cucumber, cut into matchsticks

- 2 tablespoons finely chopped red onion
- 2 tablespoons capers, drained
- 1/2 lemon, sliced thin

Instructions

- Lay a large piece of plastic wrap on a work surface.
- Arrange the slices of salmon in an overlapping fashion to create a rectangle about 6 inches wide by 12 inches long, with one of the longest sides facing you.
- Gently spread the cream cheese over the salmon trying not to dislodge any of the pieces. Lay the cucumber along one side of the rectangle about 1/2 inch from the edge.
- Using the plastic wrap to guide you, roll the salmon up tightly around the cucumber sticks. Refrigerate until firm at least 30 minutes.
- Using a sharp knife, cut the roll into 16 1/2-inch thick slices.
- Sprinkle with red onion and capers and serve with lemon slices.

Nutrition Info

Calories: 168 calories

Total Fat: 10g

Saturated Fat: 5g

Cholesterol: 22mg

Sodium: 898mg

Carbohydrates: 5g

Fiber: 1g

Sugar: 1.5g

Protein: 13.5g

23 Easy No-Cook Salsa Recipe

Get the chips ready for this quick and easy No-Cook Restaurant-Style Salsa recipe! In less than five minutes, you will have a delicious, healthy appetizer or snack everyone will love. It's bright, fresh and perfect for parties!

Total Time:5 minutes
Prep Time:5 minutes
Cook Time:0
4 Servings

Ingredients:

- 1/4 small onion
- 2 small cloves peeled garlic
- 1/2 jalapeño, seeded and membranes removed or leave in for spicy
- 14.5 ounce can diced tomatoes (not with basil) I use Tuttorosso
- handful cilantro
- juice of 1 lime
- 1/4 teaspoon kosher salt

Instructions

Place everything in the chopper of food processor and pulse a few times until combined and chunky. Don't over process.

Nutrition Info

Calories: 28 calories
Total Fat: 0g
Saturated Fat: 0g
Cholesterol: 0mg
Sodium: 201mg
Carbohydrates: 5g
Fiber: 1g
Sugar: 2g
Protein: 1g

24 Instant Pot Garlicky Cuban Pork

Tender shredded pork, marinated in garlic, cumin, grapefruit and lime and cooked in the pressure cooker is perfect to serve over a bed of rice, cauliflower rice or with tortillas and salsa and avocados for taco night.

Total Time:80 minutes plus marinade time
10 servings

Ingredients:

- 3 lb boneless pork shoulder blade roast, lean, all fat removed
- 6 cloves garlic
- juice of 1 grapefruit (about 2/3 cup)
- juice of 1 lime

- 1/2 tablespoon fresh oregano
- 1/2 tablespoon cumin
- 1 tablespoon kosher salt
- 1 bay leaf
- lime wedges, for serving
- chopped cilantro, for serving
- hot sauce, for serving
- tortillas, optional for serving
- salsa, optional for serving

Instructions

- PRESSURE COOKER: Cut the pork in 4 pieces and place in a bowl.
- In a small blender or mini food processor, combine garlic, grapefruit juice, lime juice, oregano, cumin and salt and blend until smooth.
- Pour the marinade over the pork and let it sit room temperature 1 hour or refrigerated as long as overnight.
- Transfer to the pressure cooker, add the bay leaf, cover and cook high pressure 80 minutes. Let the pressure release naturally.
- Remove pork and shred using two forks.
- Remove liquid from pressure cooker, reserving then place the pork back into pressure cooker. Add about 1 cup of the liquid (jus) back, adjust the salt as needed and keep warm until you're ready to eat.
- SLOW COOKER: Cut the pork in 4 pieces and place in a bowl.
- In a small blender or mini food processor, combine garlic, grapefruit juice, lime juice, oregano, cumin and salt and blend until smooth.

- Pour the marinade over the pork and let it sit room temperature 1 hour or refrigerated as long as overnight.
- Transfer to the slow cooker, add the bay leaf, cover and cook low 8 hours.
- Remove pork and shred using two forks.
- Remove liquid from slow cooker, reserving then place the pork back into slow cooker. Add about 1 cup of the liquid (jus) back, adjust the salt as needed and keep warm until you're ready to eat.

Nutrition Info

Calories: 213 calories
Total Fat: 9.5g
Saturated Fat: 0g
Cholesterol: 91mg
Sodium: 440.5mg
Carbohydrates: 2.5g
Fiber: 0.5g
Sugar: 1.5g
Protein: 26.5g

25 Blackened Scallops with Horseradish Sauce

These quick seared Blackened Sea Scallops are coated in a homemade blend of blackened seasoning, then cooked in a cast iron skillet served with a creamy horseradish sauce.

Total Time:25 minutes
Prep Time:15 minutes
Cook Time:10 minutes
4 servings

Ingredients:

- 1 tablespoon paprika
- 1/2 teaspoon cayenne (or more to taste)
- 1/4 teaspoon garlic powder
- 1 teaspoon dried thyme
- 1 teaspoon dried oregano
- 3/4 teaspoon kosher salt
- 1/8 teaspoon black pepper
- 1 tablespoons butter
- 16 large sea scallops (20 ounces) room temperature

Horseradish Cream

- 1/4 cup reduced fat sour cream
- 1 tablespoon prepared grated horseradish
- 1 tablespoon water
- 1/4 teaspoon Dijon mustard
- 1/8 teaspoon kosher salt
- black pepper, to taste

Instructions

- Preheat the oven to 350F.
- In a small bowl combine the horseradish cream ingredients and set aside.
- In another small bowl, add the paprika, cayenne, garlic powder, thyme, oregano, salt, black pepper and mix to blend. Coat the scallops on all sides with the spices.
- Heat a large heavy-bottomed pan or cast iron skillet over medium heat, and melt the butter.
- When very hot add the scallops and saute 1 minutes on each side.
- Transfer to the oven to finish cooking 4 to 5 minutes, or until the scallops are just cooked through and just opaque in the middle. (warning, you may want to open your windows, you kitchen will get smokey.) Serve with sauce.

For dairy free, use a dairy free butter and sour cream or preferred alternative.

Nutrition Info

Calories: 184 calories
Total Fat: 6g
Saturated Fat: 3g
Cholesterol: 60mg
Sodium: 400mg
Carbohydrates: 6.5g
Fiber: 1g
Sugar: 0.5g
Protein: 25g

26 Roasted Asparagus

This quick and easy recipe for oven roasted asparagus is the perfect spring side dish. This basic recipe can be seasoned many different ways; add lemon juice, garlic or shaved parmesan for variations.

Total Time:15 minutes
Prep Time:5 minutes
Cook Time:10 minutes
4 servings

Ingredients:

- 1 bunch fresh asparagus, about 18 ounces
- olive oil spray
- kosher salt, to taste
- fresh black pepper

Instructions

- Preheat oven to 400°F.
- Wash and trim hard ends off asparagus. Place in a single layer in roasting pan.
- Spray all over with olive oil and season with salt and pepper.
- Roast in oven approximately 10 minutes, or until render crisp.

Nutrition Info

Calories: 26 calories
Total Fat: 0g
Saturated Fat: 0g
Cholesterol: 0mg
Sodium: 2mg
Carbohydrates: 5g
Fiber: 2.5g
Sugar: 2g
Protein: 2.5g

27 Pork Chops with Dijon Herb Sauce

These Pork Chops with Dijon Herb Sauce are delicious!! One of the best ways to prepare pork chops in my opinion. So juicy and full of flavor!

Total Time:30 minutes
4 servings

Ingredients:

- 1 tsp butter
- 4 pork chops (22 oz with bone, fat removed), 1 inch thick, trim all visible fat
- 1/2 tsp salt
- fresh ground pepper

- 3 tbsp chopped onion
- 3/4 cup chicken stock or broth
- 1 tbsp dijon mustard
- 2 tbsp chopped, fresh herbs like parsley, chives

Instructions

- In a large skillet melt the butter over moderately low heat.
- Season the pork with salt and pepper.
- Raise heat to medium and add the chops to the pan and sauté for 7 minutes. Turn and cook until chops are browned and done to medium, about 7-8 minutes longer. Remove the chops and put in a warm spot.
- Add the onion to the pan and cook, stirring, until soft, about 3 minutes. Add the stock and boil until it reduces to 1/2 cup, about 2 to 3 minutes.
- Stir in the mustard, herbs, and 1/8 tsp pepper.
- Put the chops on a platter and pour the sauce over the meat.

Note:

Food and Wines says it is OK if the pork chops are pink in the center. Trichinosis is killed at the relatively low temperature of 150°. I use a thermometer to check the center and usually leave it until it hits 160°. (Don't overcook or they will become dry.

Nutrition Info

Calories: 180 calories
Total Fat: 5g
Saturated Fat: 2g
Cholesterol: 86.5mg
Sodium: 400mg
Carbohydrates: 1g
Fiber: 0g
Sugar: 0.5g
Protein: 29g

28 Classic Deviled Eggs

These classic deviled eggs are a great appetizer to any brunch or party and are so simple and easy to make.

Total Time:20 minutes
Prep Time:20 minutes
Cook Time:0
4 servings

Ingredients:

- 4 large hard boiled eggs, cooled and peeled
- 2 tablespoon light mayonnaise (regular for Keto)
- 1 teaspoon Dijon mustard
- paprika, for garnish

- Kosher salt and fresh black pepper, to taste
- 2 tablespoons chopped fresh chives

Instructions

- Use the Stove Top Hard Boiled Egg cooking method or the Instant Pot Hard Boiled Egg method to cook your eggs.
- Cut eggs in half lengthwise. Remove yolks and put them in a bowl.
- Add mayonnaise, mustard, salt and pepper to the yolks and mash.
- Transfer them to a plastic bag, snip the corner and pipe them into the egg whites.
- Top with chopped chives and paprika.

Nutrition Info

Calories: 96.8 calories
Total Fat: 7.5g
Saturated Fat: 2g
Cholesterol: 187mg
Sodium: 156.1mg
Carbohydrates: 1g
Fiber: 0g
Sugar: 0.3g
Protein: 6.3g

29 Zucchini Pork Dumplings

These low-carb pork dumplings, made with zucchini in place of dough are so dang good, you won't miss the carbs!

Total Time:45 minutes
4 servings

Ingredients:

- 12 ounces napa cabbage leaves, roughly chopped
- 1 teaspoon salt
- 2/3 pound ground pork
- 1 tablespoon grated fresh ginger (using a zester)
- 1/4 cup minced green onions (white and green parts), plus ¼ cup finely minced, green parts only, for serving
- 1/4 teaspoon ground white pepper
- 1½ tablespoons reduced sodium soy sauce, plus more for serving (or coconut aminos for gf, whole30, paleo)
- 1 tablespoon rice wine
- 2 teaspoons sesame oil
- 5 to 6 medium zucchini (about 1½ inches in diameter)
- Crushed red pepper flakes, for serving

Instructions

- Preheat the oven to 400 degrees.
- In a food processor, add the cabbage and pulse until finely minced. Set aside on a large, thin kitchen towel in the sink.

- Sprinkle with salt and let stand for 10 to 15 minutes.
- Wrap the cabbage up in the towel and wring out excess moisture over the sink (should eliminate about ⅓ cup of moisture). Set the cabbage aside.
- Meanwhile, wipe out the food processor and add in the pork, ginger, green onions, pepper, soy sauce, rice wine, and sesame oil and pulse to mix the ingredients well, being careful not to over-pulse. (You don't want the mixture to become paste-like.)
- Transfer to a large bowl and add the cabbage. Mix together with your hands to combine thoroughly. Set aside.
- Using a mandoline, slice the zucchini into 1/16-inch-thick strips. Set 1 strip down and then set another one down on top of it to create a cross shape. Repeat with 2 more zucchini strips on an angle to create an 8-cornered star shape.
- Spoon about 2 tablespoons of filling onto the center of the zucchini star. Bring the ends of the zucchini together, laying them over the filling.
- Flip the dumpling over so the seam side is down.
- Arrange on a baking sheet and repeat with remaining zucchini strips and dumpling filling, lining them up on the baking sheets as you go.
- You should create 18 to 20 total dumplings.
- Bake for 15 minutes, or until dumplings are firm and edges start to brown and crisp up.
- Transfer the zucchini dumplings to serving platters, and sprinkle with green onions and red pepper flakes.
- Serve with soy sauce.

Nutrition Info

Calories: 240 calories
Total Fat: 14.5g
Saturated Fat: 4g
Cholesterol: 51mg
Sodium: 616.5mg
Carbohydrates: 12g
Fiber: 2g
Sugar: 5.5g
Protein: 16g

30 Peruvian Green Sauce

Peruvian green sauce also known as Aji Verde is a spicy bright green condiment typically found in any Peruvian restaurant.

Total Time:30 minutes
Prep Time:5 minutes
Cook Time:0
27 servings

Ingredients:

- 2 tablespoons olive oil
- 1/4 cup chopped red onion
- 1/2 cup light Hellman's mayonnaise (use compliant mayo for whole30)

- 2 tablespoons white vinegar
- 4 teaspoons yellow mustard (Guldens)
- 1/2 teaspoon kosher salt
- 1/4 teaspoon freshly ground black pepper
- 3 jalapeños, roughly chopped seeded but keeping the ribs (about 1 cup/3 oz)
- 2 cups chopped fresh cilantro leaves and stems (2 oz) rinsed well
- 3 medium cloves garlic, crushed through a press

Instructions

- Saute the onion in a small skillet with 1 teaspoon of the oil until soft, 3 to 4 minutes.
- Transfer to the blender then add the remaining oil, mayo, vinegar, mustard, salt and pepper.
- Then add the chopped jalapeno, cilantro and garlic and blend on high speed until the sauce is smooth and creamy, about 30 seconds.

Nutrition Info

Calories: 22 calories
Total Fat: 2g
Saturated Fat: 0.5g
Cholesterol: 1.5mg
Sodium: 64mg
Carbohydrates: 1g
Fiber: 0.5g

Sugar: 0.5g
Protein: 0.5g

31 Chicken Shawarma Kebab Salad

This Mediterranean inspired salad is made with Grilled Chicken Shawarma kebabs served over salad with Feta and Tzatziki.

Total Time:35 minutes
Prep Time:20 minutes
Cook Time:15 minutes
4 servings,

Ingredients:

- 1 pound (2) boneless, skinless chicken thighs
- 1 tablespoons extra virgin olive oil
- Juice from 1 medium lemon
- 3 garlic cloves, minced
- 1 teaspoon cumin
- 1 teaspoon smoked paprika
- 1/4 teaspoon turmeric
- 1/4 teaspoon curry powder
- 1/8 teaspoon cinnamon
- Pinch red pepper flakes
- 1 teaspoon kosher salt
- Freshly ground black pepper, to taste

For the salad:

- 1 tablespoon olive oil
- 1 tablespoon red wine vinegar
- Kosher salt and freshly cracked black pepper
- 3 Persian cucumbers, chopped
- 1 cup (145 g) cherry tomatoes, halved
- 1/4 red onion, thinly sliced
- 1/4 cup feta (the kind that comes in brine), crumbled
- 4 cups butter lettuce, torn
- 1 cup Skinny Tzatziki (from my blog)

Instructions

- Cut the chicken thighs into 1-inch pieces.
- In a medium bowl, combine olive oil and lemon juice. Whisk until combined.
- Add the garlic, cumin, paprika, turmeric, curry powder, cinnamon, red pepper, salt and black pepper and whisk again. Pour the marinade over the chicken making sure it evenly coat (careful it will stain your fingers). Refrigerate and marinate for at least 30 minutes, up to overnight.
- Preheat an outdoor grill or indoor grill pan to medium-low heat.
- Thread the chicken pieces among 4 wooden or metal skewers, discarding the marinade in the bowl.
- Grill the chicken, turning the skewers occasionally, until golden brown and cooked through in the center, about 15 to 18 minutes.To make the salad:

- For the salad: In a medium bowl, whisk together the oil and vinegar and season with salt and pepper. Add the cucumbers, cherry tomatoes, and red onion and toss to combine.
- Divide the lettuce between 4 bowls, top with tomato salad, feta and grilled chicken. Serve with Tzaziki for dipping.

Nutrition Info

Calories: 284 calories
Total Fat: 14g
Saturated Fat: 3.5g
Cholesterol: 115mg
Sodium: 514.5mg
Carbohydrates: 11g
Fiber: 2.5g
Sugar: 4.5g
Protein: 29g

32 Skillet Taco Cauliflower Rice

This easy skillet dinner combines ground turkey taco meat with cauliflower rice topped with lettuce, avocado and salsa for an easy, low-carb weeknight meal!

Total Time:30 minutes
Prep Time:5 minutes
Cook Time:25 minutes
4 servings

Ingredients:

- 1 lb 93% lean ground turkey
- 1 1/4 tsp kosher salt
- 1 tsp garlic powder
- 1 tsp cumin
- 1 tsp chili powder
- 1 tsp paprika
- 1/2 tsp dried oregano
- 1/2 small onion, minced
- 2 tbsp bell pepper, minced
- 3/4 cup water
- 4 oz canned tomato sauce (1/2 can)
- 4 cups uncooked riced cauliflower

For the toppings:

- 4 ounces avocado (1 small)
- chopped cilantro
- 1 cup chopped lettuce
- 1/4 cup jarred salsa
- lime wedges

Instructions

- Over high heat, brown the turkey in a large skillet breaking it into smaller pieces as it cooks, about 5 minutes.
- When no longer pink add 1 teaspoon salt and the dry seasoning and mix well.

- Add the onion, pepper, water and tomato sauce and cover.
- Simmer on low for about 15 minutes.
- Remove the cover and add the cauliflower, add 1/4 teaspoon salt and cook until tender, about 8 minutes.
- Transfer to a plate and serve with avocado, lettuce, salsa and lime.

Nutrition Info

Calories: 256 calories
Total Fat: 13g
Saturated Fat: 3g
Cholesterol: 80mg
Sodium: 697.5mg
Carbohydrates: 12.5g
Fiber: 5.5g
Sugar: 4.5g
Protein: 26g

33 Chicken Salad with Lemon and Dill

This simple, healthy chicken salad is made with breast meat from a cooked rotisserie chicken, fresh lemon and dill. Fast and easy, and perfect for all diets including low-carb, keto, Whole30, Paleo and of course, Weight Watchers.

Total Time:5 minutes
Prep Time:5 minutes

Cook Time:0

3 servings

Ingredients:

- 10 1/2 ounces cooked skinless boneless chicken breasts (from 1 whole rotisserie chicken)
- 2 tablespoons fresh dill
- zest and juice of 1 lemon
- 1 tablespoon extra virgin olive oil
- 1/4 teaspoon kosher salt

Instructions

- Remove the chicken legs, wings and thighs from the rotisserie chicken and set aside for another meal.
- Remove the skin from the 2 breasts and remove the meat from the bones. Break the chicken into chunks with your hands or a knife and place into a large bowl. Add the fresh dill, lemon juice, lemon zest, olive oil and salt.
- Refrigerate until ready to eat.

Nutrition Info

Calories: 207 calories

Total Fat: 8g

Saturated Fat: 1.5g

Cholesterol: 84mg

Sodium: 167mg

Carbohydrates: 1.4g

Fiber: 0g
Sugar: 0g
Protein: 31g

34 Nut Butter

Homemade nut butter is so simple to make, just two ingredients (nuts and salt)! Simply toast the nuts then put them in the food processor. Here I made nut butter three ways; almond butter, walnut butter and pecan butter but any tree nut would work.

Total Time:35 minutes
Prep Time:25 minutes
Cook Time:10 minutes
28 Servings

Ingredients:

- 16 ounces (3 cups) raw almonds, walnuts or pecans*
- 1/4 teaspoon salt
- Optional: ½ teaspoon vanilla extract
- Optional to taste: ground cinnamon
- Optional to taste: maple syrup or honey

Instructions

- Preheat the oven to 350F. Spread the almonds, walnuts or pecans on a large, rimmed baking sheet and toast the almonds about 10 minutes, mixing halfway. (Don't let them get dark).
- Let them cool about 10 minutes when they are warm, not hot.
- Transfer the nuts to a high-speed blender or food processor. Blend until creamy, scraping down the sides as necessary. Be patient, it may seem like it will never turn to butter, but it will! It will go from clumps, to a ball against the side of the food processor (keep scraping the sides), then finally it will turn very creamy. If the mixture gets too hot, stop and let it cool down for a few minutes.
- Once the nut butter is very creamy, blend in the salt. If you wish to add additional flavors such as vanilla, cinnamon or honey, let the mixture cool, add the optional add ins and blend until creamy once again. Keep in mind, the texture will harden slightly if you add honey or maple syrup.
- Let the nut butter cool to room temperature, then transfer the mixture to a glass jar and tighten the lid. Store in the refrigerator for up to 3 to 4 weeks, or until you see any signs of spoilage.

Nutrition Info

Calories: 93 calories
Total Fat: 8g
Saturated Fat: 0.5g
Cholesterol: 0mg
Sodium: 10mg
Carbohydrates: 3.5g

Fiber: 2g

Sugar: 0.5g

Protein: 3.5g

35 Pollo in Potacchio (Braised Chicken with Tomatoes and Rosemary)

Pollo in Potacchio is an Italian braised chicken dish made with tomatoes, rosemary and garlic. The chicken cooks until it's fork tender, which is great served with pasta, noodles, spaghetti squash or polenta.

Total Time:varies

10 servings

Ingredients

- 10 skinless chicken thighs on the bone, 5 oz each
- kosher salt and fresh black pepper
- 3 – 4 small sprigs fresh rosemary
- 1 tbsp + 1 tsp olive oil
- 1 large yellow onion, finely chopped
- 4 garlic cloves, chopped
- 1 celery stalk, chopped
- 1 carrot, chopped
- pinch red pepper flakes, optional
- 2 cups Imported crushed tomatoes (Tuttoroso)
- 1/4 tsp dried marjoram
- 1/4 cup dry white wine (Omit for Whole30)
- 2 cups low sodium, fat free chicken broth
- kosher salt and fresh black pepper

Instructions

Dutch Oven

- Lightly season the chicken with salt and fresh pepper. Place a Dutch Oven or large heavy pot on medium-high heat. Add 1 tbsp oil, when hot add the chicken and sear until browned on all sides, about 6-7 minutes on each side. Transfer chicken to a dish and set aside.
- Sauté garlic and onions (and red pepper flakes if using) in remaining oil; sauté until golden, about 3 minutes, stirring occasionally. Add celery and carrots and saute on medium-low for about 2-3 minutes, until soft. Add the wine and chicken broth, scraping any caramelized bits from the bottom with a wooden spoon.
- Add tomatoes, marjoram, reduce heat to low, adjust salt and pepper to taste and simmer for 30 minutes.
- Add the chicken and rosemary to the sauce, partially cover and cook slowly on low heat for another 25 – 30 minutes, stirring occasionally, adding water if needed.

Slow Cooker:

- Start with the same directions step 1 and 2 on the stove, reducing the chicken broth to 1 cup. Transfer to the slow cooker with the remaining ingredients and cook on low for 8 hours.

Instant Pot:

- Lightly season the chicken with salt and fresh pepper. Press saute on the Instant Pot and add 1/2 tbsp oil, brown half of the chicken and sear until browned on all sides, about 6-7 minutes on each side. Transfer chicken to a dish and set aside, repeat with the remaining 1/2 tbsp oil and chicken. Set aside.
- Add remaining teaspoon oil, add garlic, onions (red pepper flakes if using) celery and carrots and saute on medium-low for about 3 to 4 minutes, until soft. Add the wine and 1 cup chicken broth, scraping any caramelized bits from the bottom with a wooden spoon.
- Add tomatoes, marjoram, adjust salt and pepper to taste and mix, return the chicken to the pot, add the rosemary to the sauce, cover and cook high pressure 30 minutes, natural release.

Nutrition Info

Calories: 221 calories
Total Fat: 7.5g
Saturated Fat: 2g
Cholesterol: 133mg
Sodium: 362mg
Carbohydrates: 6g
Fiber: 1.5g
Sugar: 3g
Protein: 29.5g

36 Easy Shredded Harrisa Chicken

These easy Harissa chicken recipe can be made in the slow cooker or Instant Pot (pressure cooker) and can be served so many different ways!

Total Time:4 hours
Prep Time:5 minutes
Cook Time:4 hours
4 servings

Ingredients:

- 1 pound boneless, skinless chicken breasts
- 1/2 teaspoon ground cumin
- 1/4 teaspoon garlic powder
- 1/2 teaspoon Kosher salt
- 1 cup mild Harissa sauce (I like Mina)
- optional, serve with Tzatziki

Instructions

Slow Cooker Instructions

- Season the chicken with the cumin, garlic powder, pinch of salt, and pepper.
- Place chicken in a slow cooker, pour the harissa over the chicken, and cover. Cook on HIGH for 2 hours or LOW 4 hours.
- Remove chicken from the slow cooker and shred with two forks.

Pressure Cooker Instructions

- Season the chicken with the cumin, garlic powder, pinch of salt, and pepper.
- Place chicken in the pressure cooker, pour the harissa over the chicken and cook high pressure 20 minutes. Quick or natural release then shred with two forks. If using frozen chicken breasts, cook 25 minutes.

Nutrition Info

Calories: 178 calories
Total Fat: 7g
Saturated Fat: 0.5g
Cholesterol: 83mg
Sodium: 651.5mg
Carbohydrates: 4g
Fiber: 4g
Sugar: 4g
Protein: 26g

37 Bacon Parmesan Spaghetti Squash

Roasted spaghetti squash with bacon and Parmesan cheese is a great way to top spaghetti squash for an easy, tasty, low-carb side dish.

Total Time:65 minutes
Prep Time:5 minutes
Cook Time:60 minutes
6 servings

Ingredients:

- 4 slices center cut bacon, sliced
- 1 medium spaghetti squash (yields 3 cups cooked)
- pinch Kosher salt
- 1 1/2 tablespoons extra virgin olive oil
- 1/2 cup course grated Parmigiano Reggiano
- fresh black pepper, to taste

Instructions

- Heat a medium skillet over medium heat.
- Add the bacon and cook until crisp, about 5 to 6 minutes. Transfer bacon to a paper towel with a slotted spoon.
- Preheat oven to 400F degrees.
- Line a baking sheet with foil. Cut the squash in half lengthwise, and use a spoon to scrape out the seeds and soft yellow strands. Lightly season with salt and pepper, place the squash face down on the baking sheet and bake for 60 to 65 minutes or until the flesh easily pierces with a fork.
- When soft, transfer to a bowl and combine with olive oil, parmesan, and bacon.

Nutrition Info

Calories: 109 calories
Total Fat: 7g
Saturated Fat: 2.5g
Cholesterol: 8.5mg

Sodium: 239mg
Carbohydrates: 5.3g
Fiber: 1g
Sugar: 2g
Protein: 6g

38 Ham and Swiss Crustless Quiche

This low-carb Crustless Ham and Cheese Quiche is light and delicious, perfect for breakfast or brunch (or even a light dinner)! Made with a leftover ham or ham steak, broccoli and Swiss Cheese.

Total Time:55 minutes
Prep Time:15 minute
Cook Time:40 minues
6 servings

Ingredients:

- cooking spray
- 1 3/4 cups diced ham steak or leftover ham (9 oz)
- 1 cup chopped steamed broccoli (fresh or frozen)
- 1 cup fresh grated Swiss cheese
- 2/3 cup 2% milk
- 1/4 cup half & half cream
- 5 large eggs
- 1/2 teaspoon kosher salt
- 1/8 teaspoon ground black pepper
- pinch of nutmeg

Instructions

- Preheat the to 350F degrees. Spray a pie dish with oil.
- Evenly spread the broccoli in the dish and top it evenly with the ham.
- Make the custard mixture by whisking together the milk, half and half, eggs, salt, black pepper, and the nutmeg.
- Pour the custard into the dish and top with Swiss Cheese.
- Bake 35 to 40 minutes, until the center is set.
- Cut the quiche into 6 pieces and serve.

Nutrition Info

Calories: 215 calories
Total Fat: 12.5g
Saturated Fat: 6.5g
Cholesterol: 193mg
Sodium: 620mg
Carbohydrates: 5g
Fiber: 1g
Sugar: 2.5g
Protein: 20g

39 Ranch Chicken Salad

This light and easy chicken salad recipe made with leftover rotisserie chicken breast meat and my homemade ranch dressing. Great for lunch and meal prep!

Total Time:15 minutes
Prep Time:15 minutes
Cook Time:0
4 servings

Ingredients:

- 1/2 cup 1% buttermilk
- 3 tablespoons mayonnaise
- 2 tablespoon fresh finely chopped chives
- 1/2 teaspoon kosher salt
- 1/4 teaspoon garlic powder
- 1/4 teaspoon onion powder
- 1/4 teaspoon dried parsley
- 1/4 teaspoon dried basil
- fresh black pepper, to taste
- 2 cups shredded boneless chicken breast, from rotisserie chicken or leftover

Instructions

- In a medium bowl combine the buttermilk, mayo, chives, salt, garlic powder, onion powder, parsley, basil and black pepper and mix.
- Add the shredded chicken and mix well. Refrigerate until ready to eat.

Nutrition Info

Calories: 167 calories
Total Fat: 9.5g
Saturated Fat: 2g
Cholesterol: 48mg
Sodium: 263mg
Carbohydrates: 2g
Fiber: 0.5g
Sugar: 2.5g
Protein: 17.5g

40 Veggie Ham and Cheese Egg Bake

Make this delicious and easy breakfast veggie ham and cheese egg bake for brunch or make it ahead for meal prep for the week.

Total Time:1 hour
Prep Time:10 minutes
Cook Time:50 minutes
12, Serving Size

Ingredients:

- olive oil spray
- 2 cups shredded reduced fat sharp cheddar (for gf, check labels)
- 1 tbsp olive oil
- 1/3 cup sliced scallions

- 5 oz sliced shiitake mushrooms
- 1/2 cup chopped red bell pepper
- 7 oz finely diced lean ham steak
- 3/4 cup diced tomatoes, seeded
- 1 cup finely chopped broccoli florets
- 7 large whole eggs
- 5 large egg whites
- 1/4 cup fat free milk
- 1/2 tsp kosher salt
- 1/4 tsp ground black pepper

Instructions

- Preheat the oven to 375°F. Spray a 9 x 13 baking dish with oil.
- Place 1 cup of cheese into the baking dish.
- Heat the oil in a large nonstick skillet over medium heat; add scallions, mushrooms and red pepper and sauté until vegetables are tender, about 5 to 6 minutes. Add the tomatoes and cook 2 – 3 minutes. Add the ham and broccoli and remove from heat. Spread evenly over the cheese mixture.
- In a large bowl combine the eggs, egg whites, milk, salt and pepper and whisk well. Slowly pour over the vegetables in the baking dish and top with remaining cheese.
- Bake until a knife inserted near the center comes out clean, 32 to 35 minutes. Let stand 8 to 10 minutes before cutting into 12 pieces.

Nutrition Info

Calories: 152 calories
Total Fat: 8g
Saturated Fat: 2g
Cholesterol: 102mg
Sodium: 385mg
Carbohydrates: 5g
Fiber: 1g
Sugar: 1g
Protein: 14g

41 Crustless Broccoli & Cheddar Quiche

Broccoli and cheese is one of my favorite quiche combinations! This low-carb Crustless Broccoli Cheddar Quiche is light and delicious, perfect for breakfast or brunch (or even a light dinner)!

Total Time:50 minutes
Prep Time:10 minutes
Cook Time:40 minutes
6 servings

Ingredients:

- cooking spray
- 3 cups chopped broccoli florets
- 1 cup grated cheddar cheese

- 2/3 cup 2% milk
- 1/4 cup half & half cream
- 5 large eggs
- 3/4 teaspoon kosher salt
- 1/8 teaspoon ground black pepper
- pinch freshly grated nutmeg

Instructions

- Preheat your oven to 350 degrees. Spray a pie dish with oil.
- Steam the chopped broccoli florets in the microwave with 1 tablespoon water until tender crisp and green but not mushy, about 2 1/2 to 3 minutes.
- Evenly spread the broccoli in the dish and top it evenly with the grated cheddar cheese.
- Make the custard mixture by whisking together the milk, half and half, eggs, salt, black pepper, and the nutmeg. Pour the custard into the dish and bake 35 to 40 minutes, until the center is set.
- Cut the quiche into 6 pieces and serve.

Nutrition Info

Calories: 174 calories
Total Fat: 12g
Saturated Fat: 6g
Cholesterol: 178mg
Sodium: 358mg
Carbohydrates: 5g

Fiber: 1.5g

Sugar: 3g

Protein: 12.5g

42 Jalapeno Popper "Nachos"

Jalapeno Poppers meet nachos in this fun, low-carb twist of two classic appetizers, perfect for sharing!

Total Time:45 minutes

Prep Time:15 minutes

Cook Time:30 minutes

8 servings

Ingredients:

- Reynolds Wrap Non-Stick Foil
- olive oil spray
- 1/2 pound 99% lean ground turkey
- 1 clove garlic, minced
- 2 tablespoons chopped onion, minced
- 1 tbsp chopped fresh cilantro
- 1/2 teaspoon garlic powder
- 1/2 teaspoon cumin powder
- 1/2 teaspoon kosher salt
- 1/2 tablespoon tomato paste
- 2 tablespoons water
- 8 jalapeno peppers, halved and seeded and membranes removed (use gloves)

- 3 ounces 1/3 less fat cream cheese
- 1 large scallions, green part only, sliced
- 1/2 ounce shredded sharp cheddar cheese

Toppings:

- 1/2 cup shredded sharp cheddar cheese
- chopped scallions and cilantro, for garnish
- 2 tablespoons sour cream plus 2 teaspoons water, for drizzling
- 1/2 cup pico de gallo
- 2 tablespoons sliced black olives

Instructions

- Preheat oven to 400F and line a large baking sheet with nonstick aluminum foil.
- Heat a medium nonstick skillet over medium heat and spray with oil. Add onion, cilantro and garlic and saute about 2 minutes, until soft. Add ground turkey, salt, garlic powder, cumin and cook meat for 4 to 5 minutes until meat is completely cooked through breaking it up with a spoon. Add the tomato paste and water, mix well and simmer on medium for about 2 to 3 minutes, remove from heat.
- Meanwhile, combine cream cheese, cheddar and scallions in a medium bowl. Using a small spoon or a spatula, spoon about 1 teaspoon of the cream cheese filling into the peppers.
- Arrange in a single layer, cut-side up close together. Bake until soft, about 12 to 15 minutes.
- Top with meat and cheese and bake until melted, about 3 minutes more.

- Remove from oven and top with pico de gallo, olives and drizzle with sour cream. Garnish with cilantro and scallions and serve immediately.

Nutrition Info

Calories: 111 calories
Total Fat: 6.5g
Saturated Fat: 3.5g
Cholesterol: 25.5mg
Sodium: 262mg
Carbohydrates: 3g
Fiber: 1g
Sugar: 2g
Protein: 10g

43 Buffalo Chicken Dip

This Slow Cooker Buffalo Chicken Dip has everything you love about buffalo wings, only made into a dip – no messy hands!

Total Time:4 hours
Prep Time:5 minutes
Cook Time:4 hours
9 servings

Ingredients:

- 2 boneless skinless chicken breasts (16 ounces)
- 4 oz 1/3 less fat cream cheese, softened (Philadelphia)
- 1 cup fat-free sour cream or Greek yogurt (I prefer sour cream)
- 1/2 cup Franks red hot sauce (or whatever hot sauce you like)
- 1/2 cup crumbled blue cheese
- 1 teaspoon white vinegar
- scallions, optional for garnish
- cut up celery sticks and carrot sticks, for dipping

Instructions

- To make the shredded chicken, place chicken in the slow cooker and add enough water or chicken broth to cover. Cook high 4 hours. Remove and shred with two forks, discard the liquid.
- Meanwhile, combine the cream cheese, sour cream, vinegar and hot sauce together until smooth. Add half of the blue cheese.
- Transfer to the slow cooker with the chicken, mixing well and return to the slow cooker, cook low 2 to 3 hours.
- Transfer to a serving dish and top with the remaining blue cheese, garnish with scallions. Serve hot.

Oven Method:

- To bake this in the oven, you can use cooked shredded chicken breast from a rotisserie chicken, then mix all the ingredients and place them in a baking dish. Bake 350F until hot, about 20 to 25 minutes.
- Instant Pot Method:

- Cook chicken covered in water or broth 15 min high pressure. Once you shred and drain set the instant pot to the slow cooker mode, combine ingredients and proceed.

Nutrition Info

Calories: 121 calories
Total Fat: 6.5g
Saturated Fat: 4g
Cholesterol: 48mg
Sodium: 707mg
Carbohydrates: 4.5g
Fiber: 0g
Sugar: 2.5g
Protein: 15g

44 Chicken Thighs with Shallots in Red Wine Vinegar (Poulet Au Vinaigre)

Lightened up this popular French chicken dish known as Poulet Au Vinaigre, which is made with chicken thighs and shallots cooked in red wine vinegar and white white.

Total Time:35 minutes
Prep Time:5 minutes
Cook Time:35 minutes
4 servings

Ingredients:

- 32 oz (8 lean and trimmed) boneless, skinless chicken thighs
- kosher salt and fresh pepper
- 1/2 cup red wine vinegar
- 1 cup chicken broth
- 1 tbsp honey
- 1 tbsp tomato paste
- 1 tsp butter
- 1 large shallot, thinly sliced (3/4 cup)
- 2 cloves garlic, thinly sliced
- 1/2 cup dry white wine
- 2 tbsp light sour cream
- 2 tbsp fresh chopped parsley

Instructions

- Season the chicken with salt and pepper.
- In a medium saucepan, combine vinegar, honey, 3/4 cup chicken broth and tomato paste. Boil about 5 minutes, until it reduces down to about 3/4 cup. Remove from heat.
- In a large skillet, melt butter over medium-low heat and add chicken. Cook on both sides, until brown, about 6-8 minutes. Remove chicken and set aside. Add the shallots and garlic to the skillet and cook on low until soft, about 5 minutes. Pour the sauce over the chicken, add the wine, remaining broth salt and pepper. Cover and simmer about 20 minutes until tender.
- Remove the chicken, add sour cream and stir into the sauce (if sauce dries up, add more broth). Boil a few minutes then return chicken to skillet. Top with fresh parsley.

Nutrition Info

Calories: 353.5 calories
Total Fat: 11.5g
Saturated Fat: 3.5g
Cholesterol: 219.5mg
Sodium: 398mg
Carbohydrates: 11g
Fiber: 0.5g
Sugar: 6.5g
Protein: 46g

45 Fish Florentine

This easy Fish Florentine recipe, made with a pan seared firm white fish served on a creamy bed of spinach feels like something you would order out in a fancy restaurant!

Total Time:20 minutes
Prep Time:5 minutes
Cook Time:15 minutes
4 servings

Ingredients:

- 4 (5 oz) thick pieces of skinless white firm fish fillet (such as grouper, bass or halibut)
- 1 tablespoons extra virgin olive oil

- 1 tablespoon salted butter
- 1 cup red bell pepper chopped
- 2 cloves garlic minced
- 9 ounces fresh baby spinach (from two bags)
- 2 ounces 1/3 less fat cream cheese (I like Philadelphia)
- ¼ cup half & half cream
- 3 tablespoons grated Parmesan cheese
- kosher salt
- fresh black pepper

Instructions

- In a large skillet over medium heat add 1/2 tablespoon of olive oil and 1/2 tablespoon of butter, red bell pepper and garlic and cook for about 4 minutes.
- Add spinach season with a pinch of salt and pepper mix until the spinach wilts down.
- Add cream cheese, half & half and parmesan cheese mix well until cream cheese is melted and resembles creamed spinach.
- Heat a separate skillet on medium high heat, add remaining oil and butter.
- Season fish on both sides with salt and pepper and place on the hot pan.
- Cook 6 minutes on first side and flip fish over and cook other side an additional 5 minutes, until cooked through and browned.
- Divide the spinach mixture on the bottom of each plate and top with piece of fish.

Nutrition Info

Calories: 351 calories
Total Fat: 16.5g
Saturated Fat: 6.5g
Cholesterol: 78mg
Sodium: 300mg
Carbohydrates: 6g
Fiber: 2g
Sugar: 2g
Protein: 43g

46 Classic Egg Salad

This classic egg salad recipe can be enjoyed for breakfast on toast, or for lunch in a wrap, over salad or in a sandwich. Sometimes, you can eat it with a spoon right out of the container!

Total Time:25 minutes
Prep Time:5 minutes
Cook Time:20 minutes
4 servings

Ingredients:

- 6 hard boiled eggs, peeled and chopped
- 3 tablespoons mayonnaise
- 1 teaspoon finely chopped red onion

- 1/4 teaspoon kosher salt
- fresh black pepper, to taste
- 1/8 teaspoon sweet paprika, for garnish
- chopped chives, for garnish

Instructions

- Combine all the ingredients and refrigerate until ready to eat.

Nutrition Info

Calories: 185 calories
Total Fat: 15.5g
Saturated Fat: 3.5g
Cholesterol: 282mg
Sodium: 215.5mg
Carbohydrates: 1g
Fiber: 0g
Sugar: 2g
Protein: 9.5g

47 Instant Pot Chicken Parmesan

This quick and easy Chicken Parmesan is the answer to your weeknight dreams!! And since it's made in the Instant Pot, it's ready in minutes!

Total Time:18 minutes
Prep Time:15 minutes
Cook Time:3 minutes
4 servings

Ingredients:

- 1 teaspoon extra virgin olive oil
- 2 garlic cloves, thinly sliced
- 1-1/2 cups prepared marinara sauce
- 3 tablespoons grated Parmesan cheese
- Freshly ground black pepper
- 4 thin chicken cutlets (12 ounces total)
- ½ teaspoon kosher salt, or more to taste
- ½ teaspoon dried oregano
- 4 ounces fresh mozzarella cheese, grated
- Chopped basil, for garnish (optional)

Instructions

- Using the sauté function (on low, if possible), heat the oil in the pressure cooker pot. Stir in the garlic and cook until just turning golden, about 2 minutes. Stir in the marinara sauce, 2 tablespoons of the Parmesan, and 1/4 teaspoon pepper.
- Increase the sauté heat to medium.
- Season the chicken with the salt, oregano, and pepper to taste. Nestle the cutlets into the sauce, overlapping as little as possible, then spoon the sauce over to cover the chicken.

- Lock the lid into place and cook on low pressure for 3 minutes. Manually release the pressure.
- Sprinkle the mozzarella and the remaining 1 tablespoon Parmesan evenly over the chicken. Cover the pot with the lid (but don't lock it on) and let it sit for 4 to 5 minutes to melt the cheese.
- Serve as is or, for deeper flavors and a little bit of crispiness, broil the cheese until golden and bubbling: Heat the broiler with a rack 4 inches from the heat source. Scoop the chicken and sauce into a greased small rimmed baking sheet, trying to keep the cheese on top. Broil until the cheese has browned, 2 to 3 minutes. Sprinkle with basil, if desired.

Nutrition Info

Calories: 248 calories
Total Fat: 11g
Saturated Fat: 4.5g
Cholesterol: 87.5mg
Sodium: 621mg
Carbohydrates: 7.5g
Fiber: 2g
Sugar: 3.5g
Protein: 29g

48 Roast Chicken with Rosemary and Lemon

Juicy, tender roasted chicken seasoned with lemon and rosemary, always a winner in my house!

Total Time:1 hour 20 minutes

Prep Time:10 minutes

Cook Time:1 hour

4 Servings

Ingredients:

- 1 (3 lb) chicken, washed and dried, fat removed
- 1/2 onion, chopped in large chunks
- 2 cloves garlic, smashed
- 1 lemon, halved
- 3 sprigs fresh rosemary
- 1 tbsp dried herbes de Provence (or dried rosemary)
- kosher salt and fresh pepper

Instructions

Heat oven to 425F.

- Season chicken inside and out with salt, pepper, and herbs de Provence.
- Squeeze half of the lemon on the outside of the chicken and stuff the remains of the lemon along with onion, garlic, rosemary sprigs inside the chicken. Transfer to a sheet pan, and tie the chicken by taking kitchen twine and plumping up the breast, then coming around with the string to lasso the legs and tie them together. Don't forget to tuck the wing tips under themselves so they don't burn.
- Roast the chicken with the feet towards the back of the oven, until the juices run clear, and internal temperature is 160°F,

about 50-60 minutes (Insert thermometer between the thickest part of the leg and the thigh).
- Let the bird rest for 10 minutes, tenting with foil before carving.
- Serve chicken, either one breast, or one thigh/drumstick, skin is optional.

Nutrition Info

Calories: 322 calories
Total Fat: 8g
Saturated Fat: 2g
Cholesterol: 177mg
Sodium: mg
Carbohydrates: 5g
Fiber: 1g
Sugar: 2g
Protein: 55g

49 Chopped Feta Salad

Chopped salad with romaine lettuce, Feta cheese, cucumbers, red onion and dill tossed with a simple red wine vinaigrette. An easy side salad to go with all your Mediterranean dishes.

Total Time:15 minutes
Prep Time:15 minutes
Cook Time:0
4 servings

Ingredients:

- 8 cups chopped romaine lettuce
- 1/2 English cucumber, peeled and diced in large chunks
- 1/3 cup Feta cheese, crumbled
- 1/8 small red onion, sliced lengthwise
- 1/4 cup olive oil
- 2 tablespoon red wine vinegar
- 1 1/2 tablespoons fresh chopped dill
- 1/2 teaspoon kosher salt
- fresh black pepper, to taste

Instructions

- Toss all the ingredients together and serve right away.

Nutrition Info

Calories: 173 calories
Total Fat: 16.5g
Saturated Fat: 3.5g
Cholesterol: 11mg
Sodium: 289mg
Carbohydrates: 4.5g
Fiber: 2g
Sugar: 2.5g
Protein: 4g

50 Ranch Chicken Salad

This light and easy chicken salad recipe made with leftover rotisserie chicken breast meat and my homemade ranch dressing. Great for lunch and meal prep!

Total Time:15 minutes
Prep Time:15 minutes
Cook Time:0
4 servings

Ingredients:

- 1/2 cup 1% buttermilk
- 3 tablespoons mayonnaise
- 2 tablespoon fresh finely chopped chives
- 1/2 teaspoon kosher salt
- 1/4 teaspoon garlic powder
- 1/4 teaspoon onion powder
- 1/4 teaspoon dried parsley
- 1/4 teaspoon dried basil
- fresh black pepper, to taste
- 2 cups shredded boneless chicken breast, from rotisserie chicken or leftover

Instructions

- In a medium bowl combine the buttermilk, mayo, chives, salt, garlic powder, onion powder, parsley, basil and black pepper and mix.
- Add the shredded chicken and mix well. Refrigerate until ready to eat.

Nutrition Info

Calories: 167 calories

Total Fat: 9.5g

Saturated Fat: 2g

Cholesterol: 48mg

Sodium: 263mg

Carbohydrates: 2g

Fiber: 0.5g

Sugar: 2.5g

Protein: 17.5g

51 Low Carb Potato Salad

A low-carb faux "potato" salad made with cauliflower instead of potatoes, perfect for Keto or if you're just looking to eat less carbs.

Total Time:35 minutes

Prep Time:10 minutes

Cook Time:25 minutes

6 servings

Ingredients:

- 1 pound cauliflower florets, chopped into 1/2 inch pieces
- Kosher salt
- 1/2 cup olive oil mayonnaise (I love Sir Kensington)
- 1 teaspoon yellow mustard
- 1 ½ teaspoon fresh dill
- Freshly ground black pepper, to taste
- 1/4 cup finely chopped dill pickle
- 1 medium celery stalk, finely chopped
- 1/4 cup chopped red onions
- 1 tablespoon pickle juice
- 6 hard boiled eggs, sliced
- paprika, for garnish

Instructions

- Place 1 inch of water in a large pot with 1 teaspoon salt and bring to a boil. Add the cauliflower and cook until tender, 8 to 10 minutes. Drain and set aside in a large bowl.
- Meanwhile, in a small bowl, combine the mayonnaise, mustard, dill, pinch of salt and pepper. Set aside.
- Chop 4 of the eggs and add to the bowl with the cauliflower. Slice the remaining two eggs for topping.
- Add pickle, celery, 1/4 teaspoon salt, pepper, and red onion. Add the mayo mixture and pickle juice to the cauliflower and toss gently to evenly coat. Garnish with remaining sliced eggs and sprinkle with paprika.

Nutrition Info

Calories: 222 calories
Total Fat: 20g
Saturated Fat: 3.5g
Cholesterol: 206mg
Sodium: 289.5mg
Carbohydrates: 5.5g
Fiber: 2g
Sugar: 2g
Protein: 8g

52 Shrimp Scampi Foil Packets

Shrimp Scampi Foil Packets are so fast and easy, perfect to make all summer long!

Total Time:20 minutes
Prep Time:10 minutes
Cook Time:8 minutes
4 Servings

Ingredients:

- Reynolds Wrap Heavy-Duty Aluminum Foil
- 4 garlic cloves, 2 grated, 2 thinly sliced
- 1/2 teaspoon kosher salt
- 1 tablespoons extra virgin olive oil

- 40 jumbo peeled and deveined shrimp (slightly over 1 pound)
- 1/4 cup dry white wine
- 1 tablespoon fresh lemon juice
- 4 pinches red pepper flakes
- 2 tablespoons unsalted butter, melted
- 3 tablespoons chopped parsley
- whole wheat crusty bread, optional for serving
- 1 lemon, cut into wedges

Instructions

- Whisk the grated garlic, salt, oil in a medium bowl. Add shrimp, toss to coat, and chill, uncovered, at least 30 minutes and up to 1 hour.
- Make foil packets. Tear off 4 16" sheets of Reynolds Wrap Heavy-Duty Aluminum Foil.
- Place 10 shrimp on the center of each foil sheet. Top each with remaining garlic slices, 1 tablespoon wine, lemon juice, pinch red pepper flakes and 1/2 tablespoon melted butter over each.
- Bring up the long sides of the foil, so the ends meet over the food. Double fold the ends, leaving room for heat to circulate inside. Double fold the two short ends to seal the packet
- Grill over high heat, 8 minutes. Use gloves or tongs to remove and carefully open. Top with chopped parsley. Serve with lemon wedges.
- (To bake in the oven, preheat oven to 425F and cook about 10 minutes.)

Nutrition Info

Calories: 224 calories
Total Fat: 11g
Saturated Fat: 4.5g
Cholesterol: 188mg
Sodium: 312mg
Carbohydrates: 6g
Fiber: 1.5g
Sugar: 0g
Protein: 24g

53 Grilled Lobster Tails with Herb Garlic Butter

Grilled Lobster Tails topped with Herb Garlic Butter are a delicious delicacy, and grilling them is super quick and easy!

Total Time:30 minutes
Prep Time:20 minutes
Cook Time:10 minutes
4 Servings

Ingredients:

- 4 medium lobster tails, if frozen thawed
- olive oil spray
- pinch salt and pepper, to taste
- lemon wedges, for serving

- 2 tablespoons Herb Garlic Butter (see below)

Compound Butter:

- 8 tablespoons unsalted butter (1 stick), at room temperature
- 1/4 cup (not packed) minced fresh herbs (Italian parsley, chives or basil)
- 2 tablespoons minced garlic
- 1/2 teaspoon kosher salt
- 1 teaspoon lemon zest
- 1 teaspoon lemon juice
- Reynolds Kitchens Quick Cut Plastic Wrap

Instructions

- For the butter: Place butter in a mixing bowl and use a rubber spatula to soften until it is very spreadable. Add remaining ingredients, and mix until thoroughly combined.
- Place compound butter on the center a sheet of a sheet of plastic wrap or parchment paper. Shape into a round log, and twist the ends to seal. Place butter in the refrigerator to harden, at least 30 to 60 minutes. Once solid, it will be easy to slice.
- For the Lobster: Place each tail, shell side up, on a cutting board. Using a large sharp knife, cut through the shell directly down the center, beginning at the tail and down to where the body use to be.
- Season the exposed meat with pinch of salt and fresh cracked black pepper, to taste and spritz with olive oil.
- Preheat grill to medium high, clean and oil the grates. To cook, place each tail half directly on the grate flesh side down and close the hood. Cook about 1 1/2 minutes, then turn 45 degrees (to cross-hatch), close the hood and grill for another 1 1/2 minutes.

- Remove the tails to a pan and spread each one with 1/2 tablespoon of butter.
- Return the tails to the grill, flesh side up. Close the hood and allow them to grill for another 3 to 5 minutes depending on the size, until the tail meat is opaque and firm to the touch.
- Remove the tails, serve with lemon wedges.

Nutrition Info

Calories: 177 calories
Total Fat: 6.5g
Saturated Fat: 3.5g
Cholesterol: 230mg
Sodium: 752.5mg
Carbohydrates: 0.5g
Fiber: 0g
Sugar: 0g
Protein: 28g

54 Steamed Mussels with Piri Piri Sauce

Steamed mussels get a kick with spicy Piri Piri Sauce which is basically a kicked up chimichurri sauce.

Total Time:26 minutes
Prep Time:20 minutes
Cook Time:6 minutes
4 servings

Ingredients:

For the sauce:

- 6 tablespoons finely chopped red onion
- 1/4 cup finely chopped parsley
- 3 tablespoons olive oil
- 2 tablespoons red wine vinegar
- 1 tablespoon water
- 1 garlic clove, minced
- 1/2 jalapeno pepper, seeded and minced
- 1/4 teaspoon kosher salt
- 1/8 teaspoon black pepper
- 1/8 to 1/4 teaspoon crushed red pepper

For the mussels:

- 2 pounds fresh live mussels
- 3/4 cup white wine (use broth for whole30)
- 3/4 cup water

Instructions

- Combine all the sauce ingredients in a medium bowl and mix well. Sit at room temperature while preparing the mussels.
- Place mussels in a colander and rinse them under cold water to remove any sand. Scrub them with a stiff brush under cold running water to remove any sand. The shells will be closed

until you cook them, discard any cracked shells. To debeard, use your fingers to firmly pull out the hairy filaments.

- Clean off the outsides with a brush to remove any barnacles or dirt.
- Place 3/4 cups of water and 3/4 cup of white wine in a large pot and bring to boil. Add the mussels, cover and steam until the mussels all open, 5 to 6 minutes. Carefully drain water and divide in 4 bowls.
- Top the mussels with the Piri Piri and enjoy!

Nutrition Info

Calories: 274 calories
Total Fat: 18g
Saturated Fat: 1.5g
Cholesterol: 36mg
Sodium: 723.5mg
Carbohydrates: 7g
Fiber: 0.5g
Sugar: 1g
Protein: 13.5g

55 Chicken Club Lettuce Wrap Sandwich

Chicken Club Lettuce Wrap Sandwich, a low-carb (keto) lunch idea that replaces a wheat wrap for a lettuce wrap. Just 5 ingredients, and less than 10 minutes to make!

Total Time:10 minutes
Prep Time:5 minutes
Cook Time:5 minutes
1 serving

Ingredients:

- 1 head iceberg lettuce, cored and outer leaves removed
- 1 tablespoon mayo (I love Sir Kensington) (check labels for W30)
- 3 ounces (about 6 slices) organic chicken or turkey breast
- 2 strips center cut bacon, cooked and cut in half (check labels for W30)
- 2 thin slices tomato
- 1 piece of parchment paper, about 14" x 14"

Instructions

- Place the parchment paper down on your work surface.
- Layer 6 to 7 large leaves of lettuce in the middle of parchment paper so that you create a lettuce base about 9 inches by 10 inches.
- Spread the mayo in the center of the lettuce wrap.
- Layer with the chicken or turkey, bacon and tomato.
- Starting with the end closest to you, roll the lettuce wraps jelly roll style using the parchment as your base as tight as possible.
- Halfway through rolling, tuck the ends of the wraps towards the middle.
- Continue to roll the lettuce wrap, keeping it as tight as possible and using the parchment paper to guide you.

- When it is completely wrapped, roll the remainder of the parchment around the lettuce tightly.
- Using a serrated knife, cut the lettuce wrap almost completely, leaving a small piece of the parchment intact to help hold it together.

Nutrition Info

Calories: 274 calories
Total Fat: 17g
Saturated Fat: 3.5g
Cholesterol: 73mg
Sodium: 375mg
Carbohydrates: 4.5g
Fiber: 1.5g
Sugar: 2g
Protein: 26g

56 Italian Chopped Salad

Italian Chopped Salad is my favorite quick lunch I love to whip up with ingredients I usually have on hand in my refrigerator! So simple, and can easily be modified to suit your taste.

Total Time:15 minutes
Prep Time: 15 minutes
Cook Time:0
2 servings

Ingredients:

- 4 cups chopped romaine
- 1/2 cup peeled English cucumber, cubed
- 1/2 cup halved cherry tomato
- sliced red onion
- 2 tablespoons olive oil
- 1 tablespoon red wine vinegar
- kosher salt and black pepper
- 1/2 roasted red pepper (in water), chopped
- 1 ounce genoa salami, sliced
- 6 tablespoons shredded part-skim mozzarella

Instructions

- Toss the lettuce, cucumbers, tomatoes, red onion with oil and vinegar, season with salt and pepper to taste.
- Top with roasted red pepper, salami and mozzarella.

Nutrition Info

Calories: 271 calories

Total Fat: 22g

Saturated Fat: 5.5g

Cholesterol: 22.5mg

Sodium: 556mg

Carbohydrates: 9g

Fiber: 3g

Sugar: 3.5g

Protein: 12g

57 Grilled Clams in Foil

Grilled clams cooked in foil packets with zucchini and tomatoes in a garlic white wine sauce – so fast and easy, perfect to make all summer long!

Total Time:15 minutes
Prep Time:5 minutes
Cook Time:10 minutes
2 servings

Ingredients:

- Reynolds Wrap Heavy-Duty Aluminum Foil
- 10 ounce (1 medium) zucchini, cut 1-inch pieces
- 5 cherry tomatoes, halved
- 1 clove garlic, sliced
- 3 teaspoons extra virgin olive oil
- kosher salt and black pepper, to taste
- 20 littleneck or cherrystone clams
- 1 tablespoon dry white wine (omit for Whole30)
- crushed red pepper flakes, optional

Instructions

- Preheat the grill to high heat.
- Make foil packets. Tear off 2 18" sheets of Reynolds Wrap Heavy-Duty or Non-Stick Aluminum Foil.

- In a medium bowl combine the zucchini, tomatoes, garlic, 2 teaspoons of the olive oil, 1/4 teaspoon salt and black pepper to taste.
- Place 10 clams on the center of each foil sheet. Divide the vegetables, then top with crushed red pepper flakes. Drizzle the remaining 1/2 teaspoon oil over each and 1/2 tablespoon wine over both.
- Bring up the long sides of the foil, so the ends meet over the food. Double fold the ends, leaving room for heat to circulate inside. Double fold the two short ends to seal the packet tight, so no steam escapes.
- Grill covered over high heat, until the clams open, 8 to 10 minutes. Use gloves or tongs to remove and carefully open. Eat right away!
- (To bake in the oven, preheat oven to 425F and cook about 10 minutes.)

Nutrition Info

Calories: 219 calories
Total Fat: 8g
Saturated Fat: 1g
Cholesterol: 40mg
Sodium: 878mg
Carbohydrates: 13g
Fiber: 2.5g
Sugar: 2.5g
Protein: 22.5g

58 Za'atar Lamb Chops

Grilled lamb loin chops seasoned with Za'atar, a Mediterranean blend of sumac, thyme, sesame and salt.

Total Time:15 minutes
Prep Time:5 minutes
Cook Time:10 minutes
4 servings

Ingredients:

- 8 lamb loin chops, trimmed (about 3.5 oz each bone-in)
- 3 cloves garlic, crushed
- 1 teaspoon extra-virgin olive oil
- 1/2 fresh lemon
- 1 1/4 teaspoon kosher salt
- 1 tbsp Za'atar
- fresh ground pepper, to taste

Instructions

Grill or Broil Method:

- Rub the lamb chops with oil and garlic.
- Squeeze the lemon over both sides, than season with salt, zatar and black pepper.

- Grill on an outdoor grill or indoor grill pan over medium-high heat to desired liking, about 4 to 5 minutes on each side or broil in the oven on the top rack, 4 to 5 minutes on each side.

Air Fryer Method:

- Rub the lamb chops with oil and garlic.
- Squeeze the lemon over both sides, than season with salt, zatar and black pepper.
- Preheat the air fryer to 400F. In batches in an even layer, cook to desired liking, about 4 to 5 minutes on each side.

Nutrition Info

Calories: 206 calories
Total Fat: 8g
Saturated Fat: 3g
Cholesterol: 91.5mg
Sodium: 441.5mg
Carbohydrates: 1.5gFiber: 0.5g
Sugar: 0.5g
Protein: 29g

59 Salsa Verde

A fresh, healthy salsa made with roasted tomatillos, peppers, garlic, onion and cilantro. Perfect for dipping your tortilla chips into or used in recipes that call for jarred Salsa Verde.

Total Time:30 minutes
Prep Time:10 minutes
Cook Time:20 minutes
7 servings

Ingredients:

- 3/4 lb tomatillos, husks removed
- 1 poblano chilli
- 1 serrano chili (or jalapeno for milder)
- 1 clove garlic, crushed
- 2 tbsp chopped onion
- 2 tbsp chopped cilantro
- 1/4 teaspoon sugar
- 1 tsp kosher salt

Instructions

- Preheat the broiler. Rinse and dry the tomatillos. Line a broiler pan with foil and arrange the tomatillos on the foil along with the poblano and serrano chill peppers. Broil until they are charred on top, about 3 minutes. Use tongs to turn and broil the other sides until charred, 3 to 4 minutes.
- Wrap the tomatillos and chillies in foil and let them rest for 10 minutes. Unwrap the tomatillos and chillies and peel the skin off the poblano chilli and remove the seeds. The tomatillos and serrano chilli don't need to be peeled or seeded.

- Place the tomatillos and chillies into the bowl of a food processor. Add the garlic, sugar and salt. Pulse the mixture until the ingredients are coarsely chopped.
- Add 5 to 6 tablespoons of water, the onion, and cilantro. Pulse quickly until a coarse puree forms then transfer the salsa to a serving dish. Makes about 1 3/4 cup.

Nutrition Info

Calories: 20 calories
Total Fat: 0.5g
Saturated Fat: 1g
Cholesterol: 0mg
Sodium: 161mg
Carbohydrates: 4g
Fiber: 1.2g
Sugar: 2.3g
Protein: 0.5g

60 One Pan Parmesan-Crusted Chicken with Broccoli

This simple Parmesan-Crusted Baked Chicken Breast is made on a sheet pan with broccoli, for a one pan dish that is so quick, and the best part, easy clean up!

6 servings

Ingredients:

- 2 tablespoons olive oil
- 6 (7-ounce) boneless, skinless chicken breasts
- 12 ounces fresh or frozen broccoli florets
- 1 teaspoon Kosher Salt
- 1/4 tsp garlic powder
- 2 garlic cloves, minced
- ½ cup freshly grated Parmesan cheese
- ¼ cup chopped fresh parsley

Instructions

- Preheat the oven to 425°F. Grease a rimmed baking sheet with 1 tablespoon of the olive oil.
- Arrange the chicken breasts in the center of the prepared baking sheet. Arrange the broccoli around the chicken.
- Drizzle the broccoli with the remaining 1 tablespoon olive oil and sprinkle everything with salt and garlic powder.
- Bake until the chicken breasts are cooked through and a thermometer inserted in the thickest part registers 160°F, 25 to 30 minutes.
- In a small bowl, combine the garlic, Parmesan, and parsley.
- Top each chicken breast with some of the mixture. Broil until the cheese is melted and the broccoli is deeply browned, 3 minutes.
- Remove the pan from the oven, tent with foil, and let rest for 5 minutes. Serve warm.

Freezer Friendly:
- Let the cooked dish cool completely.
- Portion it into freezer containers and freeze for up to 3 months.
- To serve, thaw in the refrigerator overnight.
- Reheat in a 325°F oven until warmed through 20 minutes.

Nutrition Info

Calories: 334 calories

Total Fat: 12.5g

Saturated Fat: 3.5g

Cholesterol: 152mg

Sodium: 448mg

Carbohydrates: 4g

Fiber: 2g

Sugar: 0.1g

Protein: 51g

61 Grilled Chicken Salad with Strawberries and Spinach Recipe

Grilled Chicken Salad with Strawberries and Spinach is made with creamy goat cheese and a white balsamic dressing, but this would also be great with Feta cheese and if you want to add more protein, or skip the cheese add walnuts or slivered almonds.

Total Time:20 minutes

4 Servings

Ingredients:

For the dressing:

- 3 tbsp golden balsamic vinegar
- 3 tbsp extra virgin olive oil
- 1 tbsp chopped shallots
- 1 teaspoon honey
- 1 teaspoon water
- 1/8 teaspoon kosher salt
- fresh black pepper, to taste

For the chicken:

- 16 oz boneless skinless chicken breast
- 1 clove garlic, crushed
- 1 teaspoon seasoned salt, to taste (I used Montreal Steak Grill Mates)

For the Salad:

- 6 cups baby spinach
- 3 cups sliced strawberries
- 2 ounces soft goat cheese

Instructions

- In a small bowl whisk together the dressing ingredients.
- For the chicken: Season chicken with seasoned salt, then mix in crushed garlic.
- Light the grill or indoor grill pan on medium heat, when hot spray the grates with oil and grill the chicken about 10 to 11 minutes on each side until charred on the outside and cooked through in the center. Set aside on a cutting board and slice on an angle.
- In a large bowl toss the spinach with the dressing. Divide between 4 plates and top with strawberries, goat cheese and
- grilled chicken.

Nutrition Info

Calories: 331 calories

Total Fat: 17g

Saturated Fat: g

Cholesterol: 89.5mg

Sodium: 345mg

Carbohydrates: 4g

Fiber: 4g

Sugar: 10.5g

Protein: 31g

62 Goat Cheese Herb Omelet with Lox

This Goat Cheese Herb Omelet topped with Nova Lox, sliced tomatoes and capers satisfies my bagel-and-lox craving, without the bagel! SO quick, takes about 5 minutes to make!

Total Time:5 minutes
1 Serving

Ingredients:

- cooking spray
- 2 large eggs
- 1 tablespoon chopped chives, plus more for garnish
- 1/8th tsp salt and pepper, to taste
- 1/2 ounce crumbled goat cheese,
- 2 thin slices heirloom tomato
- 1 ounce sliced Nova Lox
- a few sliced sliced red onion
- 1/2 tbsp capers, drained
- a few parsley leaves

Instructions

- In a small bowl beat the eggs, chive, add salt and pepper.
- Heat a medium nonstick skillet over medium-low heat. Spray with oil and pour the eggs. Cook until they set, about 2 to 3 minutes then top with goat cheese, then transfer to a plate. Top with sliced tomato, lox, red onion, capers, parsley and chives.

Nutrition Info

Calories: 239 calories
Total Fat: 15g
Saturated Fat: g
Cholesterol: 390mg
Sodium: 813mg
Carbohydrates: 3.5g
Fiber: 0.5g
Sugar: 1g
Protein: 21.5g

63 The Best Enchilada Sauce Recipe

This is hands down, The Best Enchilada Sauce Recipe ever! You'll never buy canned again!

Total Time:15 minutes
Prep Time:5 minutes
Cook Time:10 minutes
16 servings

Ingredients:

- 1/2 tsp olive oil
- 4 garlic cloves, minced
- 1 -1/2 cups reduced sodium chicken or vegetable broth
- 3 cups canned tomato sauce

- 2 tablespoons chipotle chilis in adobo sauce, chopped (to taste)
- 1 tsp Mexican hot chili powder (or more to taste)
- 1 tsp ground cumin
- 1/2 teaspoon kosher salt
- fresh black pepper, to taste

Instructions

- Heat a saucepan over medium heat, add the oil and garlic; sauté until golden, about 1 minute.
- Add the chicken broth, tomato sauce, chipotle chiles, hot chili powder, cumin and salt and pepper, to taste.
- Bring to a boil then reduce the heat to low and simmer, uncovered for 7-10 minutes.
- Set aside until ready to use. Makes 4 cups.

Nutrition Info

Calories: 21 calories
Total Fat: 0.5g
Saturated Fat: 0g
Cholesterol: 0mg
Sodium: 355mg
Carbohydrates: 4g
Fiber: 1g
Sugar: 2g
Protein: 1g

64 Turkey Enchilada Stuffed Poblanos Rellenos

These baked Turkey Enchilada Stuffed Poblanos Rellenos are peppers stuffed with a flavorful ground turkey filling, topped with my homemade enchilada sauce and cheese.

Total Time:1 hour 30 minutes
Prep Time:10 minutes
Cook Time:1 hour 20 minutes
4 servings

Ingredients:

For the poblanos:

- 4 large fresh poblano chiles
- 1 1/4 cups homemade enchilada sauce
- 1/2 cup Colby-Jack shredded cheese blend
- cilantro sprigs or chopped scallions, for garnish

For the turkey:

- 12 oz 93% lean ground turkey
- 1/4 cup onion, finely chopped
- 2 cloves minced garlic
- 1/2 medium tomato, chopped
- 1/4 cup bell pepper, finely chopped
- 2 tbsp cilantro
- 2 oz canned tomato sauce

- kosher salt
- fresh ground pepper
- 3/4 tsp ground cumin
- 1/8 tsp oregano
- 1 bay leaf

Instructions

To roast the peppers:

- Lay the poblano peppers on a work surface so they sit flat naturally without rolling.
- Using a small, sharp knife, cut a lengthwise slit along one side of each of the poblano peppers, then make a small cross-wise slit along the top to create a T-shaped slit, careful not to cut the stem off. Carefully cut out and remove the core, then scoop out the seeds.
- Using tongs, roast the poblano chiles over an open flame such as the grill, broiler or stovetop, turning often until the skin is completely blistered.
- Transfer to a plastic bag (or place in a bowl and cover with plastic wrap) and let steam for 10 to 15 minutes to loosen the skins. Once they are cool enough to handle, use a butter knife to scrape away the charred skins and discard, careful not to tear the peppers.
- Set the roasted poblanos aside.
- Preheat the oven to 350°F.
- Pour 1-1/4 cups of the sauce into the bottom of a 9 x 12-inch casserole dish.

To make the turkey:

- Meanwhile, brown the ground turkey on medium heat in large sauté pan and season with salt and pepper. Use a wooden spoon to break the meat up into small pieces.
- Add the chopped onions, garlic, pepper, tomato and cilantro and continue cooking on a low heat.
- Add cumin, oregano, bay leaves, and more salt if needed. Add tomato sauce and 1/4 cup of water and mix well, reduce heat to low and simmer covered about 15 minutes.
- Carefully stuff about 1/2 cup of the turkey mixture into each poblano pepper.
- Place the peppers seam side up over the sauce in the baking dish and top each with 2 tbsp of cheese.
- Cover the dish tightly with foil and bake in the oven until hot and bubbly, about 30 minutes.
- Serve hot topped with cilantro or scallions on top.

Nutrition Info

Calories: 233 calories
Total Fat: 5g
Saturated Fat: 5g
Cholesterol: 77.5mg
Sodium: 390mg
Carbohydrates: 13g
Fiber: 3g
Sugar: 5g
Protein: 22g

65 Enchilada Chicken Roll-Ups

These Enchilada Chicken Roll-Ups give you authentic enchilada flavor without all the work, calories or fat. And you won't even miss the tortillas!

Total Time:55 minutes
Prep Time:10 minutes
Cook Time:45 minutes
6 servings

Ingredients:

- 1 teaspoon cumin
- 2 teaspoon dried oregano
- 1 teaspoon garlic powder
- 1/2 teaspoon chili powder
- 1 teaspoon Kosher salt
- Freshly ground black pepper, to taste
- Cooking spray
- 1 (10-ounce) can mild red enchilada sauce (I used my homemade enchilada sauce)
- 1 ½ pounds (3) boneless, skinless chicken breasts, cut in half lengthwise
- 1 (4-ounce) can mild green chilis
- 1 cup reduced fat shredded Mexican cheese blend
- 1 large (6-ounce) avocado, cubed
- Chopped cilantro (for garnish)

Instructions

- Preheat oven to 375 degrees.
- In a small bowl, combine the cumin, oregano, garlic powder, chili powder, salt and pepper. Rub on both sides of each chicken piece.
- Spray a small (8×6-ish) oval or rectangular baking dish with cooking spray and pour a thin layer of enchilada sauce on the bottom of the dish.
- Lay chicken, cut side up on a work surface. Top each piece, in the center, with about 2 teaspoons chilis and 1 1/2 tablespoons cheese.
- Roll each one up and set them seam side down in the baking dish. Top with remaining sauce, cheese and chilis.
- Cover with foil and bake for 30 minutes. Remove foil and continue to bake 10-15 minutes more, or until chicken is cooked through.
- Top each chicken roll-up with a few avocado pieces and cilantro and serve.

- To freeze, transfer to a freezer safe container once cooked and cool for up to 3 months.

Nutrition Info

Calories: 261 calories
Total Fat: 11.5g
Saturated Fat: 3.5g
Cholesterol: 83mg
Sodium: 658mg

Carbohydrates: 8g

Fiber: 3g

Sugar: 1g

Protein: 31g

66 Taco Stuffed Zucchini Boats

These low-carb stuffed turkey taco zucchini boats are so easy, a fun twist on taco night!

Total Time:1 hour 15 minutes

Prep Time:15 minutes

Cook Time:1 hour

4 servings

Ingredients:

- 4 medium (32 ounces) zucchinis, cut in half lengthwise
- 1/2 cup mild salsa
- 1 lb 93% lean ground turkey
- 1 tsp garlic powder
- 1 tsp cumin
- 1 tsp kosher salt, or to taste
- 1 tsp chili powder
- 1 tsp paprika
- 1/2 tsp oregano
- 1/2 small onion, minced
- 2 tbsp bell pepper, minced
- 4 oz can tomato sauce
- 1/4 cup water

- 1/2 cup reduced fat Mexican blend shredded cheese
- 1/4 cup chopped scallions or cilantro, for topping

Instructions

- Bring a large pot of salted water to boil. Preheat oven to 400°F.
- Place 1/4 cup of salsa in the bottom of a large baking dish.
- Using a small spoon or melon baller, hollow out the center of the zucchini halves, leaving 1/4-inch thick shell on each half.
- Chop the scooped out flesh of the zucchini in small pieces and set aside 3/4 of a cup to add to the taco filling, (squeeze excess water with a paper towel) discarding the rest or save to use in another recipe.
- Drop zucchini halves in boiling water and cook 1 minute. Remove from water.
- Brown turkey in a large skillet, breaking up while it cooks. When no longer pink add the spices and mix well.
- Add the onion, bell pepper, reserved zucchini, tomato sauce and water. Stir and cover, simmer on low for about 20 minutes.
- Using a spoon, fill the hollowed zucchini boats dividing the taco meat equally, about 1/3 cup in each, pressing firmly.
- Top each with 1 tablespoon of shredded cheese. Cover with foil and bake 35 minutes until cheese is melted and zucchini is cooked through.
- Top with scallions and serve with salsa on the side.

Nutrition Info

Calories: 269 calories
Total Fat: 11.5g

Saturated Fat: 4.5g

Cholesterol: 87.5mg

Sodium: 764.5mg

Carbohydrates: 16.5g

Fiber: 5g

Sugar: 7g

Protein: 29g

67 Lobster Cobb Salad

A classic Cobb salad with a light summer twist. If you live on the coast like me and have access to fresh lobster, this salad is a must! If you're worried about cooking a live lobster, many seafood stores will steam it for you. Crab or shrimp would also make an excellent substitution.

Total Time:20 minutes

Prep Time:20 minutes

Cook Time:0 minutes

2 servings

Ingredients:

- 10 oz cooked, chilled lobster meat (yield from 2 – 1-1/2 lb lobsters)
- 2 cups baby greens
- 2 ounces avocado, diced
- 2 hard boiled eggs, sliced

- 4 slices center cut bacon, cooked and crumbled
- 1/2 cup quartered grape tomatoes
- 1/2 cup *cooked corn kernels (from 1 fresh cobb)

For the vinaigrette:

- 1 tsp dijon mustard
- 4 tsp olive oil
- 2 tbsp plus 1 tsp red wine vinegar
- 1/4 teaspoon kosher salt
- 2 tablespoons chopped red onion

Instructions

- Combine the first 4 ingredients for the vinaigrette in a small bowl and whisk well, add onions and set aside.
- Cut the lobster into large chunks. Place 1 cup greens in each bowl and top with lobster, avocado, eggs, bacon, tomatoes and corn. Drizzle 2 1/2 tbsp vinaigrette over each salad and enjoy.

You can microwave the corn 3 minutes, grill 5 minutes or cook in boiling water for about 5 minutes.

Nutrition Info

Calories: 416 calories
Total Fat: 23.6g
Saturated Fat: g
Cholesterol: 398mg

Sodium: 1171mg
Carbohydrates: 8g
Fiber: 3.4g
Sugar: 1.7g
Protein: 41g

68 Chicken and Mushrooms in a Garlic White Wine Sauce

Chicken and Mushrooms in a Garlic White Wine Sauce is a great-tasting, 20-minute dish, perfect for busy weeknights! We like it served with brown rice, pasta, quinoa or farro on the side, or a serve it with roasted veggies and a salad.

Total Time:30 minutes
Yield: 8 tenderloins

Ingredients:

- 8 chicken tenderloins, 16 oz total
- 2 tsp butter
- 2 tsp olive oil
- 1/4 cup all-purpose flour* (use rice flour for gluten free, omit for paleo, w30)
- 3 cloves garlic, minced
- 12 oz sliced mushrooms
- 1/4 cup white wine (omit for w30, paleo and add more broth)
- 1/3 cup fat free chicken broth
- salt and fresh pepper to taste
- 1/4 cup chopped fresh parsley

Instructions

- Preheat oven to 200°F.
- Season chicken with salt and pepper. Lightly dredge in flour.
- Heat a large skillet on medium heat; when hot add 1 tsp butter and 1 tsp olive oil.
- Add chicken to the skillet and cook on medium heat for about 5 minutes on each side, or until chicken is no longer pink.
- Set aside in a warm oven.
- Add additional oil and butter to the skillet, then garlic and cook a few seconds; add mushrooms, salt and pepper stirring occasionally until golden, about 5 minutes.
- Add wine, chicken broth, parsley; stir the pan with a wooden spoon breaking up any brown bits from the bottom of the pan. Cook a few more minutes or until the liquid reduces by half.
- Top the chicken with the mushroom sauce and serve.

Nutrition Info

Calories: 217 calories
Total Fat: 7.5g
Saturated Fat: 2g
Cholesterol: 88mg
Sodium: 108.5mg
Carbohydrates: 6g
Fiber: 1.5g
Sugar: 2g
Protein: 29.5g

69 BLT Lettuce Wraps

Skip the bread and enjoy all the flavors you love in a BLT, without all the carbs! So easy and seriously satisfies my BLT cravings. Add some avocado if you wish!

Total Time:10 minutes
Prep Time:10 minutes
Cook Time:0
1 Serving

Ingredients:

- 4 slices center cut bacon, cooked and chopped
- 1 medium tomato, diced
- 1 tbsp light mayonnaise (or whole30 approved mayo)
- 3 large iceberg lettuce leaves
- fresh cracked pepper
- 1 ounce avocado optional (add 1 point)

Instructions

- Carefully remove 2 large outer leaves of a head of lettuce. If you rip or tear one, just save it for the 3rd leaf you need to shred. Shred the 3rd leaf and set aside.
- Dice tomato and set aside in a bowl.
- Combine diced tomato with mayonnaise and fresh black pepper.
- Place lettuce cups on a plate, top with shredded lettuce. Add tomato then bacon and roll it like a wrap and dig in!

Nutrition Info

Calories: 161 calories
Total Fat: 10g
Saturated Fat: 2.5g
Cholesterol: 20mg
Sodium: 505mg
Carbohydrates: 8g
Fiber: 2g
Sugar: 1g
Protein: 11g

70 Chicken Pesto Bake

This easy Baked Pesto Chicken is a fast chicken dish made with skinless chicken breasts, pesto, tomatoes, mozzarella and Parmesan cheese. You can make this in the oven, or make it outside on the grill!

Total Time:30 minutes
4 Servings
Ingredients:

- 2 (16 oz total) boneless, skinless chicken breasts
- kosher salt and fresh pepper to taste
- 4 teaspoons Skinny Basil Pesto
- 1 medium tomatoes, sliced thin
- 6 tbsp (1.5 oz) shredded mozzarella cheese
- 2 teaspoons grated parmesan cheese

Instructions

- Wash chicken and dry with a paper towel. Slice chicken breast horizontally to create 4 thinner cutlets. Season lightly with salt and fresh pepper.
- Preheat the oven to 400° F. Line baking sheet with foil or parchment if desired for easy clean-up.
- Place the chicken on prepared baking sheet. Spread about 1 teaspoon of pesto over each piece of chicken.
- Bake for 15 minutes or until chicken is no longer pink in center. Remove from oven; top with tomatoes, mozzarella and parmesan cheese. Bake for an additional 3 to 5 minutes or until cheese is melted.
- To Grill: Grill chicken over medium flame on both sides until cooked through in the center. Lower flame, top chicken with pesto, tomatoes and cheese, and close grill until cheese melts.

Nutrition Info

Calories: 205 calories
Total Fat: 8.5g
Saturated Fat: 2.5g
Cholesterol: 90.5mg
Sodium: 171.5mg
Carbohydrates: 2.5g
Fiber: 0.5g
Sugar: 0g
Protein: 30g

71 Grilled Steak With Tomatoes, Red Onion and Balsamic

One of my favorite ways to make grilled steak in the summer is topped with fresh chopped tomatoes, red onion, balsamic and oil. It's fresh and a great way to enjoy those end-of-summer tomatoes!

Total Time:30 minutes
8 servings

Ingredients:

- 2 lb flank or london broil steak
- kosher salt and fresh pepper
- garlic powder
- 1 tbsp extra virgin olive oil
- 2 tbsp balsamic
- 1/3 cup red onion, chopped
- 3-4 tomatoes, chopped (about 3 1/2 cups)
- 1 tbsp fresh herbs such as oregano, basil or parsley

Instructions

- Pierce steak all over with a fork. Season generously with salt, pepper and garlic powder and set aside about 10 minutes at room temperature.
- In a large bowl, combine onions, olive oil, balsamic, salt and pepper. Let onions sit a few minutes with the salt and balsamic to mellow a bit. Combine with tomatoes and fresh herbs and adjust seasoning if needed.

- Heat grill or broiler on high heat. Cook steak about 7 minutes on each side for medium rare or longer to taste. Remove from grill and let it rest on a plate for about 5 minutes before slicing.
- Slice steak thin on the diagonal; top with tomatoes and serve.

Nutrition Info

Calories: 198 calories
Total Fat: 9g
Saturated Fat: 3g
Cholesterol: 78mg
Sodium: 71mg
Carbohydrates: 3g
Fiber: 0.5g
Sugar: 0.5g
Protein: 25g

72 Grilled Garlic and Herb Chicken and Veggies

This Garlic and Herb Grilled Chicken and Veggie recipe checks off all the boxes – quick, easy, delicious and low-carb!

Total Time:20 minutes
6 servings

Ingredients:

- 1 1/2 lbs boneless, skinless thin sliced chicken cutlets

- 3 ounce package Delallo garlic and herb veggie marinade
- kosher salt
- 1 lb asparagus (1 bunch), tough ends removed
- 1 medium 8 ounce zucchini, sliced 1/4-inch thick
- 1 medium yellow squash, sliced 1/4-inch thick
- 1 red bell pepper, seeded and sliced into strips
- olive oil cooking spray

Instructions

- Shake marinade well. Season chicken with 1/2 teaspoon salt and 2 tablespoons of the veggie herb marinade at least 1 hour, or as long as overnight.
- Marinate the veggies with the remaining marinade.
- Heat a grill over medium-high, be sure grates are clean and well oiled to prevent sticking.
- Put veggies on 1 large grill tray or 2 smaller trays (or cook in batches), season with 3/4 teaspoon salt and black pepper and cook, turning constantly until the edges are browned, about 8 minutes. Set aside on a platter.
- Cook the chicken about 4 to 5 minutes on each side, until grill marks appear and the chicken is cooked though, transfer to a platter with the veggies and serve.

Nutrition Info

Calories: 290 calories
Total Fat: 16g
Saturated Fat: g
Cholesterol: 83mg

Sodium: 145mg

Carbohydrates: 8g

Fiber: 3g

Sugar: 3.5g

Protein: 28.5g

73 Buffalo Brussels Sprouts with Crumbled Blue Cheese

These Brussels sprouts start in the skillet and finish in the oven for perfectly charred edges, then drizzled with buffalo hot sauce and crumbled blue cheese – SO good!!

Total Time:20 minutes

Prep Time:5 minutes

Cook Time:15 minutes

Ingredients:

- 2 tbsp olive oil
- 1 lb brussels sprouts, trimmed and halved
- 1/4 cup Franks Hot Sauce
- 2 tbsp crumbled blue cheese, for topping

Instructions

- Preheat oven to 425°F. Heat an oven-safe nonstick 12-inch sauté pan over medium-high heat and add olive oil and brussels sprouts in one layer and let cook undisturbed for about 3 minutes until beginning to caramelize. Turn occasionally for an additional 2-3 minutes until golden all over.

- Transfer to the oven and roast for 8-10 minutes, until softened a bit but still slightly al dente. Drizzle with hot sauce, toss and top with crumbled blue cheese.

Nutrition Info

Calories: 123 calories
Total Fat: 8g
Saturated Fat: 2g
Cholesterol: 3mg
Sodium: 657mg
Carbohydrates: 10g
Fiber: 4g
Sugar: 2.5g
Protein: 5g

74 California Spicy Crab Stuffed Avocado

These avocados are stuffed with lump crab, cucumbers and spicy mayo topped with furikake and drizzled with soy sauce. I've had this idea in my head all week, I wasn't exactly sure how it would come out but I'm obsessed with them, they came out so good!

Total Time:10 minutes
Prep Time:10 minutes
Cook Time:0
2 servings

Ingredients:

- 2 tablespoons light mayo (I used Hellmans) *for whole30 use compliant mayo
- 2 teaspoons sriracha, plus more for drizzling
- 1 teaspoon chopped fresh chives
- 4 oz lump crab meat
- 1/4 cup peeled and diced cucumber
- 1 small Hass avocado (about 4 oz avocado when pitted and peeled)
- 1/2 teaspoon furikake (I like Eden Shake or use sesame seeds)
- 2 teaspoons gluten-free soy sauce (coconut aminos for whole30/paleo)

Instructions

- In a medium bowl, combine mayo, sriracha and chives.
- Add crab meat and cucumber and chive and gently toss.
- Cut the avocado open, remove pit and peel the skin or spoon the avocado out.
- Fill the avocado halves equally with crab salad.
- Top with furikake and drizzle with soy sauce.

Nutrition Info

Calories: 194 calories
Total Fat: 13g
Saturated Fat: 2g
Cholesterol: 60mg

Sodium: 746mg

Carbohydrates: 7g

Fiber: 4g

Sugar: 1g

Protein: 12g

75 Instant Pot Chicken Cacciatore

Chicken Cacciatore made in an Instant! The sauce is hearty and chunky, loaded with chicken, tomatoes, peppers and onions (sometimes I add mushrooms too!) Great over pasta, squashta, rice or polenta.

Total Time:35 minutes

4 servings

Ingredients:

- 4 chicken thighs, with the bone, skin removed
- kosher salt and fresh pepper to taste
- olive oil spray
- 1/2 can (14 oz) crushed tomatoes (Tuttorosso my favorite!)
- 1/2 cup diced onion
- 1/4 cup diced red bell pepper
- 1/2 cup diced green bell pepper
- 1/2 teaspoon dried oregano
- 1 bay leaf
- 2 tablespoons chopped basil or parsley for topping

Instructions

- Season chicken with salt and pepper on both side.
- Press saute on the Instant Pot, lightly spray with oil and brown chicken on both sides a few minutes. Set aside.
- Spray with a little more oil and add onions and peppers. Sauté until soften and golden, 5 minutes.
- Pour tomatoes over the chicken and vegetables, add oregano, bay leaf, salt and pepper, give it a quick stir and cover.
- Cook high pressure 25 minutes; natural release.
- Remove bay leaf, garnish with parsley and serve over pasta, squasta or whatever you wish!

Nutrition Info

Calories: 133 calories

Total Fat: 3g

Saturated Fat: 0.5g

Cholesterol: 57mg

Sodium: 273mg

Carbohydrates: 10.5g

Fiber: 1g

Sugar: 5g

Protein: 14g

76 Philly Cheesesteak Stuffed Portobello Mushrooms

It doesn't get much better than a low-carb, Philly Cheesesteak Stuffed in a Portobello Mushroom! Steak and mushrooms work so well together, so why not make stuff them with this cheesy deliciousness!

Total Time:30 minutes
4 servings

Ingredients:

- 6 ounces thin sliced sirloin steaks
- 1/8 teaspoon kosher salt
- black pepper to taste
- cooking spray
- 3/4 cup diced onion
- 3/4 cup diced green pepper
- 1/4 cup light sour cream
- 2 tablespoons light mayonnaise
- 2 oz light cream cheese, softened
- 3 oz shredded mild provolone cheese (or cheese of your choice)
- 4 medium portobello mushrooms, with no cracks

Instructions

- Preheat the oven to 400F. Spray a baking sheet with oil.
- Gently remove the stems, scoop out the gills and spray the tops of the mushrooms with oil, season with 1/8 tsp salt and fresh pepper.

- Season steak with salt and pepper on both sides.
- Spray a large skillet with cooking spray and heat on high, let the pan get very hot then add the steak and cook on high heat about 1 to 1 1/2 minutes on each side, until cooked through.
- Transfer to a cutting board and slice thin, set aside.
- Reduce the heat to medium-low, spray with more oil and saute onions and peppers 5 to 6 minutes, until soft.
- Combine all the ingredients in a medium bowl. Transfer to the mushroom caps, about 1/2 cup each.
- Bake in the oven until the cheese is melted and the mushrooms are tender, about 20 minutes.

Nutrition Info

Calories: 256 calories
Total Fat: 16g
Saturated Fat: 8.5g
Cholesterol: 26.5mg
Sodium: 383.5mg
Carbohydrates: 10g
Fiber: 4g
Sugar: 3.5g
Protein: 19g

77 Chicken and Shrimp Laap

This chicken and shrimp laap or larp is a Laotian version of lettuce wraps. It's low-carb, Paleo-friendly, Whole 30 approved, loaded with flavor and so fast and easy to make!

Total Time:30 minutes
Prep Time:10 minutes
Cook Time:20 minutes
4 servings

Ingredients:

- 1 teaspoon coconut flour
- 1 teaspoon oil
- 1 small shallot, thinly sliced
- 1 pound ground chicken thighs
- ½ pound large shrimp, peeled and chopped coarsely
- 2 tablespoons Asian fish sauce
- 2 tablespoons fresh lime juice
- ½ teaspoon cayenne pepper
- 2 scallions, thinly sliced
- ¼ cup chopped cilantro
- ¼ cup minced fresh mint leaves
- 1 head butter lettuce, washed and spun dry, and separated into leaves

Instructions

- On a parchment-lined baking tray, toast the coconut flour in a 300°F oven for 5 to 7 minutes or until the flour turns golden brown. (You can also toast the coconut flour in a dry pan over low heat instead.) Set aside.

- In the meantime, heat the oil in a large skillet over medium-high heat. Add the sliced shallot and sauté for 2 to 3 minutes or until softened.
- Add the ground chicken, and break it up with a spatula. Cook, stirring, for 3 to 5 minutes until no longer pink.
- Add the shrimp and stir-fry for another 2 to 3 minutes or until the shrimp is cooked through.
- Remove the pan from the heat and add the fish sauce, lime juice, toasted coconut flour, and cayenne pepper. Adjust the seasoning to taste.
- Sprinkle the chopped herbs on top. To eat, wrap a 1/3 cup of laap in a lettuce leaf and devour.

Nutrition Info

Calories: 220 calories

Total Fat: 6.5g

Saturated Fat: 1.5g

Cholesterol: 68mg

Sodium: 795mg

Carbohydrates: 5g

Fiber: 1.5g

Sugar: 2g

Protein: 34g

78 Buffalo Brussels Sprouts with Crumbled Blue Cheese

These Brussels sprouts start in the skillet and finish in the oven for perfectly charred edges, then drizzled with buffalo hot sauce and crumbled blue cheese – SO good!

Total Time:20 minutes
Prep Time:5 minutes
Cook Time:15 minutes
4 Servings

Ingredients:

- 2 tbsp olive oil
- 1 lb brussels sprouts, trimmed and halved
- 1/4 cup Franks Hot Sauce
- 2 tbsp crumbled blue cheese, for topping

Instructions

- Preheat oven to 425°F. Heat an oven-safe nonstick 12-inch sauté pan over medium-high heat and add olive oil and brussels sprouts in one layer and let cook undisturbed for about 3 minutes until beginning to caramelize. Turn occasionally for an additional 2-3 minutes until golden all over.
- Transfer to the oven and roast for 8-10 minutes, until softened a bit but still slightly al dente. Drizzle with hot sauce, toss and top with crumbled blue cheese.

Nutrition Info

Calories: 123 calories
Total Fat: 8g
Saturated Fat: 2g
Cholesterol: 3mg
Sodium: 657mg
Carbohydrates: 10g
Fiber: 4g
Sugar: 2.5g
Protein: 5g

79 One Skillet Chicken with Bacon and Green Beans

This quick and easy chicken dish is cooked in a white wine sauce with string beans and bacon, all in one skillet. You can modify this basic recipe using any veggies you like!

Total Time:20 minutes
4 Servings

Ingredients:

- 4 strips center-cut bacon, chopped
- 1 pound boneless, skinless chicken breasts, cut lengthwise into thin cutlets
- kosher salt
- freshly ground black pepper

- 2 tablespoons minced shallot
- 2 cloves garlic, minced
- ¾ cup low-sodium chicken broth
- ½ cup crisp white wine, such as Sauvignon Blanc (use broth for Whole30 or Paleo)
- 1 teaspoon chopped fresh thyme
- 8 ounces French green beans

Instructions

- Heat a large non-stick skillet over medium heat. Add the bacon and sauté until brown and crisp. Remove bacon pieces with a slotted spoon, transfer to a paper towel lined plate and set aside. Discard the majority of the bacon grease, leaving a very thin coating in the pan.
- Season both sides of the chicken pieces with 1/4 tsp salt and black pepper and add to the skillet. Cook 4 minutes per side, or until cooked through. Transfer to a plate and tent with foil.
- Add the shallots to the now empty skillet and sauté 1 minute, scraping up brown bits. Add the garlic and sauté 30 seconds more. Add the broth, wine and thyme and stir. Add the green beans, increase the heat to medium-high and cook for about 8 minutes, or until the sauce has reduced and the green beans are crisp tender, stirring occasionally.
- Transfer the chicken breasts and green beans to a serving platter. Season beans with 1/8 teaspoon salt and fresh pepper. Pour chicken juices into sauce with 1/8 teaspoon salt, stir and cook for an additional 30 seconds. Pour sauce over the chicken and green beans and top with chopped bacon.

Nutrition Info

Calories: 211 calories
Total Fat: 5g
Saturated Fat: g
Cholesterol: 75mg
Sodium: 334mg
Carbohydrates: 7g
Fiber: 2g
Sugar: 1g
Protein: 29g

80 Arugula Salad with Crispy Proscuitto, Parmesan and Fried Eggs

This easy salad has all my favorite things in one – arugula, Proscuitto, shaved Parmesan and a runny egg! When you pop that egg yolk, the salad is bathed in that warm eggy goodness, salad nirvana in every bite!

2 Servings

Ingredients:

- 2 ounces sliced proscuitto (4 slices)
- 5 cups baby arugula
- 1/4 cup shaved parmesan cheese
- olive oil spray

- 2 large eggs
- fresh black pepper, to taste

Dressing:

- 2 tbsp minced shallots
- 2 tbsp extra virgin olive oil
- 1 tbsp sherry vinegar
- 2 tsp Dijon mustard
- 1/4 tsp honey

Instructions

- Preheat oven to 375°F. Line a large baking sheet with parchment paper.
- Arrange the proscuitto on the prepared baking sheet and bake 15 minutes or until lightly browned and crisp. Crumble into large pieces.
- Meanwhile, whisk the dressing ingredients in a large bowl. Add the arugula and toss well. Divide on two plates and top with crumbled proscuitto and parmesan.
- To cook the eggs heat a large nonstick skillet over medium-low heat, spray with oil and gently break the eggs. Season with salt and cook, covered until the whites are set and the yolks are still runny, or longer if desired. Place the egg on top of each salad and serve with fresh pepper, if desired.

Nutrition Info

Calories: 344 calories

Total Fat: 24g

Saturated Fat: g

Cholesterol: 216mg

Sodium: 1043mg

Carbohydrates: 8g

Fiber: 1.5g

Sugar: 4g

Protein: 18.5g

CONCLUSION

Quick weight loss plans are just temporary and sometimes risky. Keep in mind that a healthy weight loss requires patience, effort, consistency, and determination. Set realistic goals in your weight loss plan to be able to continue it with dedication. Success in losing weight is a combination of healthy diet and proper exercise.

Always remember too that it is very important to ask a health care professional for advice before starting on any weight loss diet or exercise to make sure that there are no medical issues that will be put to greater risks by doing quick weight loss programs or other short-term weight loss plans.

Made in the USA
Monee, IL
15 April 2021